Practice Nursing: Stability and Change

Margaret Damant
MPhil, BA, RGN, RHV, DN Cert, RHV Tutor Cert, FRSH
Community Health Nurse Teacher
Department of General Practice
University of Exeter
Formerly Principal Lecturer in Health Studies
Polytechnic South West (now University of Plymouth)

Constance Martin
MPhil, RGN, RM, RNT, DN Cert, Dip N, Dip ED
Nurse Advisor
East Sussex Family Health Services
Practice Nurse
Eastbourne

Sheila Openshaw
BSc, PhD, RGN, RHV
Course Organiser, MSc in Health Care:Professional Education
Department of General Practice
University of Exeter

With a Foreword by Professor George Castledine

⋈ MOSBY

Copyright © 1994 Mosby–Year Book Europe Limited
Published by Mosby–Year Book Europe Limited
Printed and bound in Great Britain by Biddles Limited, Guildford and King's Lynn

ISBN 0 7234 1882 9

A CIP catalogue record for this book is available from the British Library.

For full details of all Mosby–Year Book Europe Limited titles please write to
Mosby–Year Book Europe Limited, Lynton House, 7–12 Tavistock Square, London
WC1H 9LB, England.

Contents

Foreword

I find the most exciting thing about nursing at present is the comparison between the past, the present and the future. Furthermore, to evaluate history and to compare progress with the circumstances and effects of present-day changes and developments is a rare opportunity. To be able to do this in one book and enjoy the experience is indeed a great pleasure.

Practice nursing is no different from any other branch of nursing in that it requires the application of knowledge, the development of critical reasoning, decision making and practical skills. This inspirational book will guide practitioners, increase their knowledge and influence their approach to nursing practice issues.

Just as nursing practice must remain dynamic, sensitive, relevant and responsive to the changing needs of patients and clients, so too must the education of practice nurses. This book, written by three leading experts in the field, is certainly more than just a start towards this process.

It is a provocative, revealing and exciting book which will not only become an essential reference, but a key stimulus to those who read it.

George Castledine

Introduction

Most people are curious about the meteoric rise of practice nursing and the position it has established within the primary health care team (PHCT), outside the traditional line management structure of the NHS.

Practice nurses are well known for their belief that they are 'different from community nurses'. To some extent they are right because of their close relationship within the 'family' of general practice. Generally speaking, whilst the other branches of community nursing have developed relatively independently of general practice, practice nursing has developed from within general practice.

This book analyses the process. It traces the historical development and the professionalisation of nursing in general practice. It examines the scope of nursing within general practice, the expertise which is available and those aspects which need to be developed to meet the changing health needs of the population, in both the short and longer term.

The authors' work is guided by the principle that the needs of the patient are paramount, whilst acknowledging the need to address the escalating cost of health care within the context and discipline imposed by finite resources.

The book is written at the beginning of a period of rapid change and new challenges in health care provision and professional accountability. It is a time of transition (transformation) during which the ideals of democracy and equality are being dominated by the more pragmatic motivating influences of economic efficiency, innovation and flexibility. It is a time when the PHCT is concerned with new organisational interest, clinical development and financial incentives for good practice. This is causing the professions to examine their unique and collaborative role and the appropriateness of existing educational frameworks and practices, particularly the role of multiprofessional education.

The aims in writing this book are therefore to inspire nurses in general practice to give the best possible service within the multiprofessional team, and to open up issues for debate in order to lead nursing in general practice forward as a composite contributor to community nursing services which are central to the health of the nation.

Acknowledgements

It would be impossible to name all those to whom the authors are indebted for their help in obtaining, analysing and compiling the information to write this book. First and foremost are the practice nurses who, as a professional group, are tireless in their endeavours to establish an identity and to secure quality education and training appropriate to the needs of the practice populations they serve, and which enables them to make an effective contribution as members of a multiprofessional primary health care team. Without their energy and motivation there would not have been a book to be written.

There are, however, specific situations which have provoked our thinking. These include the work of the English National Board's review of the education and training for practice nursing and the contacts which have ensued. The East Sussex Family Health Services Authority's Practice Nurse Consensus Conference and the Department of General Practice, Exeter Practice Nurse Curriculum Development Workshops generated new concepts of nursing in general practice and its long term potential.

The same is true of the opportunity for debate and the exchange of information provided by various organisations such as the Yorkshire and West Midlands Practice Nurse Associations' Annual Conferences.

The willingness of our tutor colleagues to share their ideas and act as a sounding board was appreciated.

We feel we must make special mention of individual members of the caring professions who have encouraged our work and challenged our assumptions. We particularly acknowledge the contribution made by Professor Denis Pereira Gray, Professor of General Practice, University of Exeter. Two very experienced practice nurses made a major contribution in many different ways, Janet Ahmad from Eastbourne and Ann Hall from Exeter. We would also like to thank the reviewers who read our work with insight and for their constructive advice.

1 The historical perspective of nursing in general practice

'We can chart our future clearly only when we know the path which led to the present.'
Extract from Adlai Stevenson's speech, Richmond Va, 20 September 1952 .

The development of practice nursing has to be viewed within the context of the total scenario of social change and the movement of nursing. The pathways which have led to present day practice nursing as a profession, with clearly defined functions responding to need, have their origins in the general practice and in the professionalisation of nursing. To some extent both disciplines have progressed simultaneously but in many ways they have also developed independently of each other. The historical review traces this process in relation to the evolution of community nursing, aspects of social change, the introduction of the National Health Service, primary health care as a philosophy for clinical intervention, and the increasing autonomy of nursing in general practice.

1.1 The general practice origins of practice nursing

General practice is described as the oldest form of medical care, with its beginnings dating back to the Apothecaries Act in 1815 (Fry, 1988). The contribution of the general practitioner's (GP's) wife to the work of the practice in those early days seems to be as ingrained into the fabric of our society as that of the GP himself.

Marriage partnerships between doctors and nurses seem to have provided opportunities for an extension of life skills and parenting roles to include the practice population. An example of the GP's aura of paternalism is reflected in the self image of some GPs who felt that 'patients expect to believe in the doctor in a rather total way ... a father figure' (Haug, 1976). Because the GP's home was his base in the early days, this often single handed cottage industry relied not only on the support of his wife but when the children were old enough they played their part in answering the telephone and delivering medicines (Loudon, 1985).

The 'doctor's lady', as the GP's wife was alternatively known, acted as secretary, assistant treasurer, accountant and nurse. She was seen as the cornerstone of the practice – the first and last ancillary helper (Lane, 1969). Loudon describes the GP's wife as the original 'dragon at the gate' protecting her husband, often acting as first contact for the patients. She offered compassion and understanding to the sick and their relatives, many of whom feared hospital as Nightingale records in her Notes on Nursing (1895). Loudon suggests that the role of the GP's wife could provide an opportunity for the study of a unique phenomenon of social history, for just as the 'neophyte GP was untrained for his job, so was his wife'. Indeed, this support continues to be a key element of general practice but what has not always been recognised is that it may also be a source of stress to the doctor's family (Pereira Gray, 1982).

1.2 The evolution of community nursing

The gradual professionalisation of nursing from the pre-Nightingale era moved through contrasting periods of change, for example, the period of enlightenment when the seeds of 'community nursing' and its vocational elements were nurtured by St Vincent de Paul in Germany and France, to the 'dark ages' of the Sarah Gamps' tradition in this country as described by Dickens in his story of Martin Chuzzlewit (1844).

Nightingale was instrumental in moving nursing forward by her commitment to the proper selection and training of those who were to work as nurses and care for the sick in hospital. Nevertheless, her early ideals were slow to be established because of the hospitals' demand for 'numbers' to staff the wards, and the doctors' intention to retain the accountability of nursing to medicine (Baly, 1986).

Baly quotes Nightingale as having arrived at the conclusion that hospitals were not the best place for the poor sick ... and that the ultimate destination of all nursing of the sick is in their own homes. Nightingale, however, drew a distinction between 'sick nursing' and 'health nursing' but 'regarded both kinds as necessary to put us in the best possible conditions for nature to restore or preserve health, to prevent or to cure disease or injury' (Austin, 1957). This belief is the essence of Nightingale's Natural Law theory of Nursing (Fitzpatrick, 1989). As a consequence, Nightingale, along with other nineteenth century visionaries such as Rathbone (Stocks, 1960) and De'Ath (McEwan, 1959), made a significant contribution to the development of community nursing in this country.

It is interesting to note that during this period when general practice was establishing its identity and the foundations of practice nursing were being laid, parallel developments were taking place in community nursing as a complementary outpost. Stocks describes the establishment of the early District Nursing Associations, whose role was to set and monitor standards of practice, to provide training and to set examinations. At this stage in the history of health visiting there was no requirement for 'health missioners', as they were also known, to hold a nursing qualification. Indeed the work was often undertaken by assistant medical officers, a rather ironic similarity with the present day debate – *nurse* v. *medical assistant* (Stilwell and Hobbs, 1990).

Nightingale chose to describe the emerging discipline of preventive health care as a new role for women that was neither greater, or lesser than nursing but different. Until the Royal Society of Health assumed the responsibility for health visitor education and training in 1955 (with a remission for candidates who held a nursing qualification), preparation was provided by the voluntary organisations and/or local public health departments.

1.3 Social change in the early twentieth century

Social changes and population trends in society, particularly those which introduce new patterns of behaviour, influence cultural traditions and values and change the nature of employment and work, can affect the health of the community. Brief examples are drawn from three different aspects of social change which have directly and indirectly influenced the development of practice nursing.

The first of these examples illustrates the relationship between the economy and the health status of the population. Friendly societies and informal local Sick Clubs were the main source of funding for medical care, pre-1911. Historians have examined the limitations of these provisions using the health status of the Boer War recruits in the late nineteenth century as one of the main indicators of deprivation. It is recorded that many of these recruits were lame, deaf, illiterate, malnourished and suffered from rickets; they were often infested and suffered from untreated congenital deformities. The health status of recruits to the First World War (1914–1918) was only marginally improved. Social policy in the form of the Lloyd George Insurance Scheme introduced in 1911 was one of the measures taken to improve the health of the working population, but the scheme did not include the worker's dependants. This development increased the work of the GP and it is reported that the first practice nurse was appointed about this time (Martin, 1987).

The second example briefly illustrates the effect of an aspect of social change on the position of women. During the two World Wars, women had established themselves as an important element in the potential wealth (and defence) of the nation. They had an expectation of a continuing role in the labour force of the country, a goal which was not always sanctioned during times of economic depression. However, the introduction of compulsory education meant that women, in principle, had the chance to benefit from a higher degree of equality of opportunity with their male counterparts than hitherto. Women, albeit in small numbers and largely from the upper classes, were gaining places in the universities, they began to enter the professions and to break down the hallowed portals of the traditional male strongholds such as medicine. In 1980 it was estimated that the ratio of female:male GPs was 1 in 6, and by 1990 there had been a shift to 1 in 3 (DOH, 1992a). Two years later evidence suggested that the proportion of female GPs continues to increase (DOH, 1992b). Loudon considers the effect of this trend and speculates that whilst in the past doctors tended to marry nurses, they are now as likely to marry their female medical colleagues and form husband and wife partnerships in general practice. As a consequence one of the early features of nursing in general practice may be approaching a significant change but perhaps of more importance is that issues related to women's health could have a higher profile than hitherto.

The third example highlights the revival of holistic clinical practice. Writings about the changes taking place in the medical and allied professions suggest that the predominant interest of twentieth century is social in its orientation (Garrison, 1929). These conclusion are drawn by tracing the long period of evolution from 'primitive medicine' which Garrison regarded as 'essentially a phase of anthropology', through the era of medieval medicine and the organisation of hospitals, sick nursing, medical legislation and education. The subsequent advances of the 'Renaissance period' with the birth of anatomy as a science, and the growth of surgery as a handicraft were seen to precede eighteenth century medicine. This period also witnessed the beginnings of pathology as a science but with the added interest of preventive medicine. Jenner's work on preventive inoculation and the formulation of public health programmes are cited as examples. During this period psychologists developed measurements for the assessment of intellect and personality. Garrison paid tribute to a revival of the Greek ideal of athletics and personal hygiene. He asserted that the most noticeable trends to influence twentieth century medicine were cooperation at international level and the advancements in prophylactic health care, i.e. the means by which to prevent the occurrence, the recurrence or the spread of disease.

The prophylactic advancements, social orientation of health care and interprofessional networks to which Garrison refers are wide ranging and can clearly be seen to have influenced the preventive ethos of nursing in general practice and community care. For example:

● Environmental health and hygiene and the wider concerns of 'green' issues.
● Personal fitness, including nutrition and mental health.
● The social control of substance abuse and infectious diseases.
● The inclusion of intellectual, personality and developmental assessment as part of comprehensive health assessment and the management of subsequent intervention.
● The use of medical biographies and statistics by which the health of populations are measured and described, the scope of which has been expanded though the development of information technology.
● The formation of the Geneva Convention in 1864–1949, with its concerns for human rights and freedom in times of war and the aftermath.
● International congresses which encourage cooperation between universities and other institutions, such as the professions, expanding the network for research and facilitating debate and the exchange of information.
● The formation of the International Council of Nurses (ICN) in 1899 took place as part of an expanded professional community. The ICN aims to develop and improve the profession, its contribution to the health services and to promote the welfare of nurses worldwide (Baly, 1986). The ICN Code of Ethics for Nursing (1965) continues to represent the values of contemporary practice and strives to advance the professionalisation of nursing.

Attempts to think about nursing in a theoretical way began to develop and first principles were identified as the beginning of a scientific basis for practice (Fitzpatrick and Whall, 1989). Nightingale had always regarded the lack of a scientific basis as the Achilles heel of nursing.

1.4 The beginnings of the 'welfare state'

Nineteenth century reformers are often viewed as pragmatic rather than doctrinaire (Stern, 1966). Stern argued that despite evidence of need, it was not until the twentieth century that government took action to introduce a coherent programme of social reform, beginning with the provision of a school meals and medical service in 1906. He regarded this move as one of the first steps towards the achievement of Winston Churchill's objective 'to provide a plimsoll line below which nobody should be allowed to sink'.

The Beveridge Report continued the social debate for the prevention of illness and the promotion of health in its widest sense, and promulgated the ideology of the 'welfare state' (Beveridge, 1942). The British Medical Association (BMA) vehemently opposed the 'Beveridge Plan', whilst nursing and some of the professions allied to medicine were cautiously in favour of the development. The main tenets of the BMA's argument, as recorded at the time in the press, centred around issues of clinical freedom, the availability of resources and the ethics of socialised medicine. The BMA later retracted its opposition as a result of negotiating to contract out of the centralised service to retain their clinical freedom and managerial autonomy. GPs also bargained with the consultants to achieve the same status. The Beveridge Report resulted in a plethora of legislation which aimed to slay five malignant giants which were seen to cripple the health and welfare of the people of the United Kingdom. The five giants were disease, idleness, ignorance, squalor and want. The legislation denounced the Poor Law principle of 'less eligibility' and replaced it with the principle of 'eligibility' based on the identification of need. Although the new legislation was rooted in a rather more liberal and humanistic ethic, many saw the 'means test' associated with the proof of eligibility, as a relic of the Poor Law. Alternatively, they saw the new benefits as charity; either way it was abhorrent to many people. As a consequence, much health education was, and in some instances still is required to change attitudes in order that those with incomes below the declared poverty line might achieve a higher standard of health and quality of life. In addition to the new social welfare and benefits schemes, a growing recognition of the uniqueness of the individual was reflected in the Butler Education Act of 1944. The focus of this new process and outcome of general education changed from a commitment to the 'three Rs' – reading, 'riting and 'rithmetic, to the three As – age, aptitude and ability.

The National Health Service Act (1946), which came into operation on 5 July 1948, signalled a heightened awareness towards positive health and the patient's right to direct access to medical care. The objective of the National Health Service (NHS) was to provide preventive health care, diagnosis and treatment of illness free at the point of the delivery of care, from the cradle to the grave. The NHS was a tripartite administration in which community health and some welfare services were the responsibility of local government; the hospitals and family practitioner services were administered by separate authorities, as illustrated by the examples included in **Figure 1.1** (p. 14).

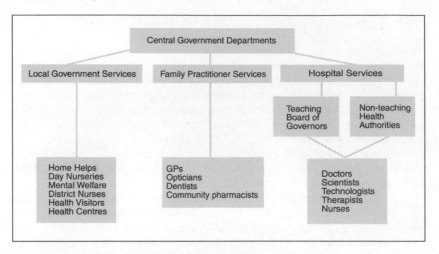

Figure 1.1 The tripartite administration of the NHS.

Arguably the most regrettable decision of all, in terms of promoting integration between the various disciplines, was not simply the creation of a third arm of administration in the form of a Family Practitioners' Committee, but that it operated in isolation from other community health services, particularly nursing. Another unfortunate facet of the new administration was the separation of health and social services within the local government sector.

The Medical Officer of Health (MOH) was designated the chief officer for the local government arm of the tripartite system and was accountable to the County Council or County Borough Council. The MOH under the terms of the NHS Act, Section 21, was charged with the responsibility of developing Health Centres. The purpose of the Health Centre was to centralise and integrate the tripartite system at the point of delivery of care. The Health Centre was seen as the means by which to achieve interprofessional liaison, quality care and a service easily accessible to the community it served. Health Centres were slow to develop. On the one hand it appeared that the different disciplines were suspicious of the power they perceived to be invested in the MOH and as a consequence they feared a 'take-over'. On the other hand it is argued that the MOH may have suffered from the low status and prestige attributed to the role by medical colleagues (Gill, 1976). Gill suggests that this situation probably resulted from a perceived lack of functional autonomy in the work place because so much of the MOH's achievement was dependent on other disciplines, e.g. environmental health. It was a relationship which continued in some areas long after the demise of the MOH and the introduction of the Community Physician in 1974.

In some respects the remnants of the conflict-ridden tripartite system still exist and many look to the Health and Social Services reforms of the 1990s to finally bury the hatchet. Meanwhile, attempts were made to maintain confidence in the NHS and its underlying philosophy. The population began to have higher expectations of health professionals, and nurses in general practice were part of this changing scene.

1.5 Primary health care: a philosophy for clinical intervention

The term primary health care has become synonymous with community, or non-institutional care. Initially the term primary care referred to medical care, the GP being the first point of contact for the patient within the health care system in the United Kingdom. The GP diagnoses and treats the patient's condition, requesting special investigations to assist diagnosis and management. Alternatively, the patient may be referred to the hospital. It is for this reason that the GP is often referred to as the 'lynch pin' of the NHS. The present day primary health care (PHC) service is a much broader concept. For example, Fry (1988) described primary professional health care as 'the first level of contact which may fall within the province of the doctor, practice nurse, medical assistant, independent nurse practitioner, social worker, or others'. This was a far-seeing notion which may be regarded to be in keeping with the views of colleagues who envisage a future when a range of different expertise could be required within the practice.

Clearly, PHC both as a concept and professional discipline has travelled (and is still travelling) a long and often tortuous road since the inception of the NHS in 1948. Fry examined the way in which general practice had moved away from the lone doctor and his wife arrangement, where the doctor's home was his work place, into an organised branch of medicine within the multiprofessional health centre setting. Some significant features can be isolated as having played a critical part in the transition of nursing from its role within this 'cottage industry' of general practice to its present position within the PHCT.

The turning point in primary care was probably the introduction of the GPs' Charter in the 1960s as both clinicians and politicians sought to redirect the role of primary health care towards the achievement of more pro-active health care goals (Gillie, 1963). The Charter was an attempt to promote teamworking between GPs, health visitors (HVs), district nurses (DNs) and other disciplines in the community. It also aimed to recognise the ancillary staffing needs of general practice and as a consequence allowed GPs to employ a full range of skills including nursing. The effectiveness of the Charter was strengthened by amendments to NHS legislation which legitimised the role of the HV and DN in general practice by expanding the sphere of professional activity to 'elsewhere, other than the home'. The Harvard Davis Report (1971) reinforced the value of such multidisciplinary groupings of health care provision directly available in a locality as a means by which the needs of the population could be met with greater sensitivity and effectiveness. Paradoxically, the statutory role of the HV ceased to be laid down in legislation (NHS Act 1968), whilst recommendations for changes in child life protection (Curtis, 1946) and the welfare of handicapped and disabled persons (Seebohm, 1968) gave a higher profile to the relatively new profession of social work. It is worthy of note that about this time the clinical and social pathology of child abuse, or the battered child syndrome was recognised and documented as a diagnosis (Kempe, 1962).

The term 'primary health care' was first formally acknowledged in the Annual Report of the DHSS, in 1974:

> The aim is to create primary health care teams in which general medical practitioners, home nurses (DNs), health visitors and in some cases social workers and dentists, work together as an inter-disciplinary team, thus facilitating coordination and mutual support in the planning and delivery of care.

The reorganisation of local authority boundaries created co-terminosity between local government and health authority boundaries. It was anticipated that this would promote a more integrated and cost-effective relationship between institutional and non-institutional care, and health care and social work (Redcliffe-Maud, 1969). In addition, to further enhance the administration and delivery of community nursing services, the traditional functional management system was replaced by a new organisational structure based on geographical multi-functional units of administration (Mayston, 1969). It might have been reasonable to assume at this stage that the scene was set for an integrated community service with flexible role boundaries also able to maximise the specialist functions of the practitioner at the point of delivery of care. This did not happen, although some health authorities promoted the participation of HVs and DNs in the services provided by the practice to which they were 'attached'. During this time nurses in general practice were quietly beavering away doing valuable work. A survey of nurses and nursing (excluding HVs and midwives) in primary medical care in England estimated that nurses in general practice represented about 20% of nurses working in the community. The findings also revealed that few nurses were the wives of GPs and even fewer were unqualified, i.e. their names were not included on any part of the Register maintained by the General Nursing Council for England and Wales (Reedy, Philips and Newell, 1976). At this time the Department recognised the training needs of practice nurses and encouraged health authorities to include them in their in-service training programmes (STM (77) 13).

It was generally recognised that members of the primary health care team (PHCT) could make a contribution to the health of the nation, for example the infectious diseases of childhood were on the decline and immunisation rates were increasing. Developmental assessment carried out by HVs on the pre-school child were identifying potentially handicapping conditions for early treatment or management. The Department recognised the dynamic quality of health care and the potential of nursing to meet the continually changing demands by extending the traditional clinical role of the nurse (HC(77)22). People were beginning to expect to survive congenital handicaps and other disabling conditions. The population as a whole had expectations of longevity. Some authorities who gave evidence to the Royal Commission on the Reform of the NHS, suggested that the concept of the PHCT was generally quite favourably accepted and that in well established, properly functioning teams a more comprehensive service was provided. Staff also seemed to obtain greater job satisfaction.

However, there were many concerns that PHC was not realising the full scope and potential of its role in improving the health of the nation. For instance, the Royal College of Nursing's (RCN) evidence to the Royal Commission argued that merely 'Pushing back the frontiers of death is not necessarily an indication of a healthier or more satisfied society'. The RCN was also concerned that PHC had 'grown up in the rough and tumble of empiricism' and the lack of research based strategic planning and practice was openly criticised. Moreover, 'teams' were seen to have come together in a haphazard way with problems of divided command, lack of accountability and cohesion which could result in tragic circumstances, such as the victims of child abuse (RCN, 1977). In addition the RCN questioned the GPs' apparent lack of accountability for public finance – the family practitioner services were seen to be 'the great planning lacuna'. A decade later, similar concerns became apparent in the Review of Community Nursing as recommendations were made for central funding of community and practice nurses (Cumberlege, 1986). The vexed question of who should employ the practice nurse caused considerable debate. Practice nurses strongly expressed a desire to retain their present employment relationship with the GP and showed great antipathy towards returning to the traditional NHS hierarchy.They also valued their close working relationship with the GP which gave them immediate access to advice and consultation. Practice nurses felt that this method of working promoted quality care and patient satisfaction (Peachey, 1987). The other side of the debate expressed concern about the way in which the employment relationship might detract from the nurse's professional autonomy within the PHCT (Clark, 1987).

The GPs' non-cash limited budget was a source of frustration to health authorities, many of whom lacked the resources to improve their community nursing manpower and patterns of working in the way they would have wished to do so, and in accordance with RCN recommendations to the Royal Commission (1977) and those of later enquiries (Acheson, 1981; Harding, 1981). Furthermore, the RCN criticised the under-use of the health centres and urged that they become centres of education and prevention as well as of treatment and consultation. At this time others were commenting on the power rituals and routines which took place in the health centre. For instance, it was seen to 'stand as a monument to popular expression of the belief that men are made, in part at least, by their environment ... with planners and participants anticipating some ensuing change in the actions, attitudes and relationships of those who work there.' (Beales, 1976). But there is little evidence to suggest that this happens. In a later publication, Beales graphically described the visit of the nursing officer to the health centre and the 'ruffled feathers' that were often left behind – an example of the bureaucracy which nurses in general practice found so abhorrent (Beales, 1978). This account is perhaps also an unwitting illustration of the RCN's concern for the disenchantment and conflict which can often be experienced within the PHCT. Social workers also reported problems of divided loyalty. Clearly, it was no coincidence that the central objective of multi-professional education was to bring the different disciplines together to encourage empathy and to gain an understanding of each other's perspectives and constraints in the achievement of better patient care (England, 1979). But another important message was beginning to emerge regarding the scientific evidence on which the PHCT was founded and whether it was necessarily the best, or only way of delivering effective preventive health care to the community. The philosophy of PHC is rarely in doubt; indeed both internationally and nationally it is continually reinforced. For instance, the World Health Organisation

(WHO), established in 1948 by the United Nations Organisation, was initially concerned with the eradication of smallpox. Over a period of time WHO became more concerned about wider concepts of health to include:

● Health as a right for all people.
● The eradication of inequalities.
● Community involvement for health.

In this regard WHO declared that:

> PHC is essential health care, based on practical, scientifically sound and socially acceptable methods and technology, made universally accessible to individuals and families in the community through their full participation and at a cost the country can afford to maintain, at every stage of their development, in the spirit of self-reliance and self-determination. It forms an integral part of the country's health care system, of which it is the central function and the main focus, and of the overall social and economic development of the community. It is the first level of contact of individuals, the family, and community with the national health system, bringing health care as close as possible to where people live and work, and constitutes the first element of a continuing care process.
>
> The Alma-Ata Declaration 1978

The promotion of health and the prevention of disease are the central elements of WHO initiatives, the scope of which has been described at various points along a continuum of primary, secondary and tertiary intervention and care. Its spectrum stretches from health (mental, physical and social) as a function of the whole fiscal–social policy, to screening for vulnerability and the early detection of presymptomatic disorder and finally to the process of damage limitation in chronic conditions (Kapnio, 1979). A later publication by the Royal College of General Practitioners (RCGP) distinguished between the prevention of disease and the promotion of health as different ways of thinking and acting, whilst each contributed to the other. The two different but complimentary activities are defined as:

● The prevention of disease to include measures which:
   – remove risks by dealing with causes.
   – limit complications, damage and disability arising from established disease.
● The promotion of health was generally regarded as that part of preventive work which is the furthest from most doctors' habits of thought and action. It was seen to entail helping people to learn and accept responsibility for their own well being (RCGP, 1981).

The English National Board for Nursing, Midwifery and Health Visiting (ENB) completed a review of education and training for practice nursing in 1990. Three elements of health care were identified, taking into account the literature, including the consumer perspective (Ong *et al.*, 1989). The three elements are set out in **Figure 1.2** .

PRIMARY HEALTH CARE

Involves healthy people, to prevent disease or disability before it occurs. It includes positively improving the quality of health and the quality of life.

For example:
Education (child and adult)
Balance of work: leisure (use of leisure facilities)
Housing/adequate shelter
Communication networks
Prevention of poverty
Accident prevention
Hygiene and waste disposal } safe
Clean water   } environment
Control of air pollution
Personal relationships
Nutrition, exercise
Stress management
Education for health

SECONDARY HEALTH CARE

Relates to the early detection and treatment of disease and involves people with previously undetected disability or disease and the restoration of good health.

For example:
Screening for hypertension, hearing tests, cervical cytology, breast/self examination, compliance with a therapeutic regime, early detection of substance abuse or its potential e.g. alcohol, smoking, drugs, food, the establishment of self care regimes.

TERTIARY HEALTH CARE

Involves action to avoid unnecessary progression or complications of permanent disease or disability.
For example:
Self care and the avoidance of complications from asthma, diabetes; control of epilepsy; rehabilitation training following accidents or disease; re-enablement of older people.

Adapted from: Ong *et al.*, 1989; Coutts and Hardy, 1985; Ewles and Simnett, 1985.

Figure 1.2 Elements of health care (Extracts from Damant, 1990, *A Review of Education and Training for Practice Nursing*).

Several different types of care in the community have been described by Fry. The first is 'self care within the family/community' and it is suggested that this form of care may deal with approximately three quarters of all episodes of illness. The second group is the 'self carers', a group which is often supported by other professionals such as nurses or therapists. This group might represent a significant proportion of the work load in general practice together with those patients/relatives who elect to consult directly with the nurse. Thirdly, there are 'those who consult with the GP', clearly a relatively small proportion of the practice population considering that it is generally estimated that the GP is consulted in only one quarter of all episodes of illness. Questions must therefore be asked about those who are unknown but ought to be screened or receiving health care, the 'submerged portion of the iceberg' (Donaldson and Donaldson, 1984). It is also this group about whom the RCN and others who gave evidence to the Royal Commission voiced concern. For example the RCN cited several surveys which demonstrated the extent of the unrecognised health needs of the population. One such survey which revealed that only 12% of the population were healthy in so far as they had been symptom free for the previous 2 weeks. The RCN, along with others seems to question the nation's ability to provide health care.

From other platforms it seemed that all may not be well with the PHC and social welfare system. The authors in preparing material for this chapter examined many sources of statistical data and found evidence of high mortality and morbidity amongst people in the lower socio-economic groups. One such publication was the Black Report in 1980 (Davidson and Townsend, 1982). The findings of the Report identified a range of adverse social conditions that appeared to be associated with ill health. These were coupled with increasing levels of unemployment and had fundamental implications for social policy and the way in which the PHCT functioned both individually and as a group. The late 1970s and early 1980s was a period of growing concern about the ability of the NHS to cope with the actual and potential health related problem. Nuttall in her address to the RCN Annual Conference highlighted the misconceptions upon which the NHS was established. For example, she drew attention to the original intention that the NHS would be funded through a situation of full employment whereby everyone would make a contribution to exchequer funds, and that once the backlog of ill health had been dealt with the costs would be reduced and the nation would become healthier (Nuttall, 1977).

Reflecting back nearly half a century and in circumstances where unemployment has been an escalating problem rather than a diminishing one, and where the demand for health care has become almost insatiable, it is tempting to ask how successful we have been in dealing with Beveridge's five giants. In the 1970s there seemed to be two arguments about the future provision of health care. On the one hand the case was for capital investment and a closer relationship between general practice and the public sector, coupled with a refocusing of professional education and the deployment of resources and technical knowledge for use in the community (Bury, 1968). On the other hand, the case was beginning to be made for increased public awareness, and the inevitability of the need to prioritise in situations where the demand for health care, and patient expectations, are not only higher but infinite.

It was not until the 1980s that the Griffiths Management Study introduced the 'commercial ethic' to health care with its implications for quality assurance and 'value for money' (Griffiths, 1983). The Report on Health Information Systems in the community demonstrated the appalling absence of substantive data for strategic planning and the audit of health care systems (Körner, 1984). The potential of the data base available within general practice was seen to represent a relatively untapped reservoir of problem identification, planning and evaluative material. The NHS as it approaches the twenty-first century and its golden anniversary must realise the full potential of this resource for strategic planning. All members of the PHCT are in a position to make full use of what Fry describes as a 'unique opportunity for long term observation and study of disease and the processes of health'. The importance of this data base for nursing in general practice should not be overlooked. The potential of this resource for targeting health needs and developing clinical practice is discussed in some detail in the following chapters.

1.6 The development of nursing in general practice

Clearly, nursing itself has developed within the developing framework of general practice and PHC resulting in specific peaks of activity and growth. The explosion of practice nursing activity which hit the press, the conference platform and the political arena was mainly due to the catalyst effect of the Cumberlege Report and its apparent lack of appreciation of the scope of the nursing role in general practice. Indeed, the way in which some practice nurses had been able to expand their role in primary, secondary and tertiary health care was a testimony to their drive, insight and creativity, and to their commitment to PHC. For example, practice nurses were showing their expertise in the screening of at-risk groups, monitoring the health of the chronically sick and teaching self care. In many instances practice nurses were offering open access to patients, making a nursing diagnosis and selecting appropriate forms of intervention. However, there is some evidence to suggest that the concepts of teamwork and networking were less well developed (Dunnel and Dobbs, 1980).

The continuing momentum of the developing role of the nurse in general practice was a feature of the 1980s (Fowler *et al.*, 1988), (Stilwell, 1985) and (DHSS Health Circulars, 1977, 1989). A review of the advertisements in the professional press for practice nurse vacancies was undertaken by the authors. This also shows a move away from the 'anyone will do attitude' such as 'Nurse/Receptionist needed to work in a doctor's surgery', to a slightly more focused approach, e.g. 'SEN or SRN required for part-time work in a busy health centre'. In recent times the advertisements have been more discerning, obviously seeking to attract professional practitioners who are well equipped to develop the full potential of the role, e.g. 'RGN, preferably PN, HV or DN qualified required to provide skilled nursing care, to establish and manage health promotion'. The introduction of the 1990 GP Contract (DOH and Welsh Office, 1990) had phenomenal implications for the professional accountability of nurses in general practice, as testified by the guidance issued by the United Kingdom Central Council for Nurses Midwives and Health Visitors (UKCC,1990). The service demands of the GP Contract created an explosion in the number of practice nurses employed and in some inner city areas severe recruitment problems were reported (Damant, 1990). There was some concern that the situation would perpetuate the wide variations in the social and occupational characteristics of practice nurses identified by earlier studies (Greenfield *et al.*, 1987). For instance, the study suggested that whilst the role of the practice nurse was developing in some practices, the majority of nurses were still confined to the 'technical tasks', and only a small minority (15%) indicated that they wished to extend their role. Nevertheless, some interesting developments can be observed from the findings. For instance, 12% of the sample were involved with research, 96% offered direct nurse consultations and nearly 90% were used to the GP asking for their professional opinion either about the management of a case, or method of treatment.

The literature and anecdotal evidence seems to suggests that three issues are central to the struggle experienced by practice nurses to develop their role and professional identity. First is the lack of appropriate training with professional and academic accreditation. This situation has been compounded by the way in which their own profession has neglected their petition for so long. Second is frequently seen to be the lack of support and encouragement given to them by their GP employers. Evidence suggests that some employers inhibit the professional development and scope of the nurse either though their lack of understanding of the nursing role, or negative attitudes to education and training (Damant, 1990). The third constraint was often attributed to the lack of commitment demonstrated by health authorities (including the Department) and the professional associations.

However, this apparent lack of interest and support was not universal; for example, some of the early practice nurse courses were instigated by the Departments of General Practice in the Universities. The introduction of a statutory requirement for vocational training for GPs encouraged these developments and fostered joint training activities between trainee GPs and practice nurse students, and between their respective trainers. Some GPs, along with the RCN facilitated the formation of local associations and interest groups which gradually linked into a national network.The enterprise of practice nurses during the 1980s was commendable. They used their interest groups and associations for peer support and professional development, and as a political platform for change. Access to the Royal College of General Practitioners (RCGP) through their GP employers strengthened the political clout of practice nurses and resulted in the establishment of a working group to examine the training needs of the practice nurse. The working group, which included representatives from the RCGP, RCN, Panel of Assessors for District Nurse Training and the Council for the Education and Training of Health Visitors, published a report and made recommendations for the future education and training of practice nurses (RCN, 1984). The Report was received with some disappointment. Firstly, it did not recommend a mandatory requirement for training, and secondly the syllabus was seen to fall short of the need for quality nursing care in general practice. To some extent it might be argued that the Report was a reflection of the different perceptions of the role and function of the nurse in general practice. The apparent polarisation of such views became evident in the press and various publications, for example 'How close has the practice nurse come to the nurse practitioner, or medical assistant?'(Stilwell and Hobbs, 1990). On the one hand this might imply that the role fell within the traditional province of medicine rather than nursing. There are models in Scandinavia and America where the medical assistant is prepared through a separate portal of entry, similar to the preparation of theatre technicians in the UK. On the other hand, the preparation of the nurse practitioner can be seen to equip the nurse to function at an advanced level of nursing practice wherever this approach is adopted, both within and outside the UK. Neither approach seemed to represent the position of nurses in general practice in the 1980s, although there are indications for a rethink as we approach the 1990s.

Meanwhile, to offer a way forward the recommendations of the working group were approved and implemented by the National Boards for Nursing, Midwifery and Health Visiting in England, Northern Ireland, Scotland and Wales conditional upon a review after a period of 3 years.

As would be anticipated, some educational institutions interpreted the recommendations in a much wider context than others. The triennial review conducted by the National Boards resulted in a broader based and more detailed analysis (Damant, 1990). The review was well received by the profession and is currently contributing to the wider debate on the future of community health nursing education and practice (UKCC, 1991).

One course evaluation produced evidence of some encouraging findings which suggested that during the course some nurses began to demonstrate a more positive attitude towards their role as a nurse (Stilwell and Drury, 1988). Fewer respondents seemed to think that their role was to save the doctor's time by merely relieving him/her of certain tasks. Many students gave a higher priority to the assessment of patients' risk factors but rather surprisingly, a lower priority was awarded to health education. The evaluation did not appear to include an assessment of teamworking skills, or the practice nurse's perception of his/her identity within the PHCT. Feedback on this apparently rather under-developed aspect of practice would have been helpful in view of the findings of the Dunnel and Dobbs survey referred to above. In addition a smaller scale study of 20 GP practices in Wales also revealed that practice nurses felt the need for more professional contact and education with their GPs and other members of the PHCT (Owen, 1978). Others have also identified the professional isolation of practice nurses and the implications for team care (Bowling, 1981; Martin, 1987). Notwithstanding the distinguishing features of nursing in general practice, practice nurses were included in a comprehensive study of community nursing, its role and practice within the PHCT in England (Cumberlege, 1986). Similar reviews were undertaken in Northern Ireland, Scotland and Wales. The four reviews all recognised the potential of this trained labour force but recognised that the self-limiting practices imposed by the profession itself were often counterproductive.

The profession was accused of being tied by 'chains of tradition' and by letting the 'warring factions distract the professionals from the opportunities to expand their role and to work in closer partnership with the patient'. The Marplan survey conducted as part of the Cumberlege review suggested a reasonable level of consumer satisfaction with the service. Some consumers indicated that in certain circumstances they would seek direct access to the community nurse in preference to the doctor. The Survey corroborated the findings of the WHICH Survey (1987) where the results clearly indicated that nursing was considered by both doctors and patients to be an essential element of PHC. However, some research suggests that there is no room for complacency; for instance in rural communities there are clear indications that all community services could be improved (Giarchi, 1989).

In future nurses in general practice will be expected to accept their responsibility to advocate for the patient by contributing to the procurement of quality health care. Clearly, PHC is not an end in itself but a means towards providing the optimum level of health care in the community. The way forward for practice nursing is as a composite part of a community nursing service.

Just as the 1940s represented a watershed for health and welfare services, the late 1980s laid the foundation for a refreshing philosophy of collaborative working in which the locus of power for health decisions was to be vested in the patient, i.e. a shift from the doctor's charter to the patient's charter (DOH, 1991) Furthermore, the promotion of health (primary, secondary and tertiary) was given a high priority in social policy and professional education (GP Contract, DOH, 1990; Project 2000, UKCC, 1986). One of the most significant assumptions underlying the new policies for health care is that practice and clinical decision making will be based on a health contract between professional(s) and the patient, the carer(s) and where appropriate, the community.

There is a requirement to utilise more effectively the entire spectrum of expertise within the PHCT through shared care and interdisciplinary team working (Caring for People, and Working with Patients, DOH, 1989) which culminated in the National Health Services and Community Care Act (1990). The potential effects of these changes are far reaching and provide a challenge to all members of the PHCT and the society they serve.

1.7 The move towards multiprofessional education for members of the PHCT

Multiprofessional education (also referred to as interprofessional education) has for over a quarter of a century been regarded as the panacea for all ills in the PHCT. This belief was reiterated by Government in its 'Programme for Improving Primary Health Care' (1987), to quote 'the best way to encourage people to work together is not clear ... but the patterns of community care are changing rapidly and teamwork is increasingly important ... there is a case for bringing the various disciplines together for at least part of their course ... although their roles will differ'. However, this may also be seen as an attempt by Government to paper over the cracks in the service rather than to address the more complex and fundamental political issues, or the limitations of the PHCT mode of delivery of health care. The Nottingham Symposium on inter-professional learning has been acknowledged to be the turning point for collaboration in education and practice (England, 1979). Although much has been achieved, there is increasingly more work to be done as teams become less motivated by ideals of democracy and equality, and more by notions of efficiency, innovation and effectiveness. In addition, there is some evidence to suggest that shared learning, or interprofessional learning does not necessarily have positive outcomes for all participants (Damant, 1991). Evidence suggests that this might be more to do with the process of education than the content (Williams, 1979; Jones, 1986; Shakespeare, 1989). On the other hand, there is some indication that multiprofessional continuing education had more successful outcomes (Ashton, 1992). Shakespeare's study shows HVs and DNs to be the two groups most frequently involved in multiprofessional education activities. Practice nurses throughout the literature are usually noticeable by their absence. However, an interesting finding from Damant's research suggests that HVs and DNs generally regard practice nurses to be a valuable component of shared educational initiatives. Such developments are vital for the cohesion and creativity of community nursing.

The Centre for the Advancement of Interprofessional Education in Primary Health Care (CAIPE) was established in 1987 and forms part of the European Network for the development of Multiprofessional Education in Health Sciences (EMPE). These organisations work to promote multidisciplinary working, education and research throughout Europe. This work will become increasingly important as a means of testing and strengthening the primary health care ethic.

The ENB Review of the education and training needs for practice nursing attempted to bridge the transitional phase for nursing in general practice at a time when numerous long term objectives were in hand. The group worked from a conceptual framework which supported the belief that practice nursing is:

● *A concept* rooted in a *value system* directed towards addressing the health needs of society by nursing within the context of general practice. Its values are implicit within the philosophy of PHC (WIIO, 1978) and the Code of Professional Conduct (UKCC, 1984); it is consistent with the ethos of the new preparation for the professional role of the nurse (Project 2000, UKCC 1986).
● *A collaborative process and an integral part of community nursing* which results in timely intervention through which individuals and their families are assisted to recovery, or to cope with the stress of illness or suffering (Travelbee, 1971).
● *A clinically based discipline* whose theory grows out of and is tested in practice; it contributes to research and uses research findings.
● *A dynamic agent for change* through the development of nursing care and patient empowerment in general practice.

As a consequence, the Review (Damant, 1990) concludes that the role and function of the nurse in general practice is underpinned by a range of complex processes as set out in **Figure 1.3**.

These processes have implications for a minimum standard of post-registration education and training with learning outcomes which respond to continually changing health care needs. They also call for a more unified and flexible approach across all spheres of practice, with the emphasis on a multi-professional framework to influence the structure, process and outcome of the learning experience.

- **Problem solving and decision making processes,** within limits of time, environment, the nature of decisions PNs are empowered to make by their employers, and their access to a varying range of resources. An ability to recognise the potential complexity of the apparently 'simple' problem and the implications of omission and commission.

- **Interpersonal processes** with the accent on rapid relationship- making skills and teamship; a counselling approach and the ability to hold constructive health conversations at different levels of complexity.

- **Professional processes,** nursing, autonomy and accountability with due regard for the rights, autonomy and individuality of the patient/client. Acting as the client's advocate/mediator.

- **Teaching and learning processes,** particularly in regard to health education, respecting the value systems and beliefs, self motivation and personal development of others.

- **Clinical processes** in which knowledge of disease processes and their treatment are paramount and where safe practice is determined by an awareness of the extended role, human caring skills and value-free judgements.

- **Health promotion and maintenance** processes underpinned by epidemiology, neighbourhood knowledge, concepts of health which take account of the ageing process and an awareness of ethical considerations.

- **Management processes** in relation to self, time and enabling resources; the effectiveness and well being of other members of the team. Marketing.

- **Research processes,** including the application of first principles of research to practice, the use of research findings, and the undertaking of research.

Figure 1.3 Processes which underpin practice nursing (Damant, 1990). (Reproduced by permission of the English National Board.)

Summary

A genealogy of the family tree of community nursing can be found in Appendix 1 (p. 117). It illustrates the convergent and divergent pathways of the three main strands of general nursing in the community (i.e. practice nursing, district nursing and health visiting), together with a selection of the various forces which have influenced the development of the professional role, its education and practice. The movement towards the present position can be traced through three distinct but accumulative phases as influenced by the work of the early environmentalists, and at a later stage by the individualistic person-focused approaches, to the present holistic, community focus of the collectivist perspective. Several trends are of interest, notably:

- Nightingale as a major influence.
- The non-nursing origins of health visiting.
- District nursing as a source from which other specialisms have emerged.
- The rise and decline of specialisms synonymous with health trends and social forces.
- The longer pre-professional stage of practice nursing.
- The re-conceptualisation of community nursing as a composite entity.
- The move towards multiprofessional activities as the concept of team working matured.
- A shift in the locus of control from 'profession' to 'consumer'.

The experience of compiling the family tree of community nursing might be likened to that of a visitor who asked a 'local' the way to a certain place. After considerable thought the 'local' replied 'Of course, I would not have started from here, but since you are going to have to ...'.

History suggests that practice nursing has moved through three phases of professionalisation. The first was the transition from the doctor's wife to practice nurse following the introduction of statutory registration and the protection of the title of Nurse as a safeguard for the general public. A second stage from practice nurse to practice nursing emerged from the ENB Review which concentrated on the processes of practice nursing. Finally, based on current trends and evidence of the untapped potential of the nursing contribution to PHC, we have identified a third transition from practice nursing to nursing in general practice. The following chapters address this process.

References

Acheson E D (1981), *Report of a Study Group 'Primary Health Care in Inner London'*. London: Health Planning Consortium

Ashton J (1992), *The Evaluation of a Multi-Professional Scheme of Continuing Education*. Unpublished PhD Thesis. University of Exeter.

Austin A L (1957), *History of Nursing Source Book*. New York: Putman's and Sons.

Baly M E (1986), *Florence Nightingale and the Nursing Legacy*. London: Croom Helm.

Beales G (1976), Practical sociological reasoning and the making of social relationships among health centre participants. In Stacey M (ed) *The Sociology of The National Health Service.* University of Keele, pp. 61–75.

Beales G (1978), *The Sick Health Centre.* London: Pitman Medical Press.

Beveridge W (1942), *Report of the Committee on Social Insurance and Allied Services.* London: HMSO.

Bowling A (1981) *Delegation in General Practice. A Study of Doctors and Nurses.* London: Tavistock Publications.

Bury HS (1968), A Health Service for Tomorrow. *The Medical Officer of Health,* Diamond Jubilee Number, 29 November, pp. 316–317.

Clark J (1987), Practice Nurses A GP Employee? The Case Against. *Nursing Times,* April 29, **83**(17), p 35.

Coutts LC and Hardy LK (1985) *Teaching for Health.* London: Churchill Livingstone.

Cumberlege J (1986), *Report of the Community Nursing Review 'Neighbourhood Nursing – A Focus for Care'.* London: HMSO.

Curtis M (1946), *Report of the Care of Children Joint Committee.* London: HMSO.

Damant M (1990), *Report of the Review Group for the Education and Training for Practice Nursing 'The Challenges of Primary Health Care in the 1990s'.* London: English National Board for Nursing, Midwifery and Health Visiting (ENB).

Damant M (1991), *A Comparative Study of Shared Learning between Health Visitors and District Nurses.* Unpublished MPhil thesis. University of Plymouth.

Davidson M and Townsend P (1982), *Inequalities in Health.* London: Penguin.

DHSS HC (77) 22. *The Extending Role of the Clinical Nurse. Legal Implications and Training Requirements.* (Ref also PL/CNO (89)10).

DOH (1989), *Caring for People: A Review of Care in the Community.* London: HMSO.

DOH (1989), *Working for Patients: A Review of the National Health Service.* London: HMSO.

DOH PL/CMO (89)7 & PL/CNO (89) 10. *The Extending Role of the Nurse.* DOH.

DOH (1990), *The National Health Service and Community Care Act.* London: HMSO.

DOH (1991), *The Patients' Charter.* London: HMSO.

DOH (1992) *Statistics for General Medical Practice in England and Wales 1980– 1990.* DOH Statistical Bulletin 4(2). London: HMSO.

DOH (1992) *General Medical Services Basic Statistics in England and Wales.* Oct 1. London: HMSO

DOH and Welsh Office (1990), *Terms and Conditions for Doctors in General Practice.* The NHS (General Medical and Pharmaceutical Services) Regulations 1974 Schedules 1–3 as amended.

Donaldson R J and Donaldson L J (1984), *Essential Community Medicine.* Lancaster: MPT Press Ltd.

Dickens C (1844), *Martin Chuzzlewit.* London: Oxford Press.

Dunnel K and Dobbs J (1980), *Nurses Working in the Community.* London: OPCS.

England H (1979), Education for Co-operation in Health and Social Work. *Journal of the Royal College of General Practitioners,* Occasional Paper 14.

Ewles L and Simnett I (1985), *Promoting Health.* London: John Wiley and Sons Ltd.

Fitzpatrick J J and Whall A (1989), *Conceptual Models of Nursing: Analysis and Application.* 2nd edn. East Norwalk CT: Appleton and Lange.

Fowler G, Fullard E and Gray JA (1988), The Extended Role of the Practice Nurse in Preventive Health Care. In Bowling A and Stilwell B (eds) *The Nurse in Family Practice: Practice Nurses and Nurse Practitioners in Primary Health Care.* London: Scutari, Ch 8.

Fry J (1988), *General Practice and Primary Health Care 1940–1980s.* London: Nuffield Provincial Trust.

Garrison G (1929), *History of Medicine.* Philadelphia: W B Saunders Co.

Giarchi G G (1989), *Deprivation in a Cornish Setting.* London: NACAB.

Giarchi G G (1989), *Information Deprivation in a Rural Setting*. London: NACAB.
Gill D G (1976), The Reorganisation of the National Health Service. In Stacey M (ed) *The Sociology of the NHS*. University of Keele, pp. 9–23.
Gillie A (1963), *Report of a Sub-Committee of the Central Health Services Council 'The Work of the Family Doctor'*. (The GPs' Charter) London: HMSO.
Greenfield S, Stilwell B and Drury M (1987), Practice Nurses: Social and Occupational Characteristics. *Journal of the Royal College of General Practitioners,* **37**(301), pp. 341–345.
Griffiths R (1983), *National Health Services Management Enquiry*. London: DHSS.
Harding W G (1981), *A Report of a Joint Working Group of the Standing Medical Advisory Committee and the Standing Nursing and Midwifery Advisory Committee 'The Primary Health Care Team'*. London: DHSS.
Harvard Davis (1971), *A Report of the Sub-Steering Committee of the Standing Medical Advisory Committee 'The Organisation of Group Practice'*. London: HMSO.
Haug M R (1976), Issues in General Practitioner Authority in the National Health Service. In Stacey M (ed) *The Sociology of the NHS*. University of Keele, pp. 23–42.
International Council of Nurses (1965), *Code of Ethics*. Geneva.
Jones R V H (1986), Working Together – Learning Together. *Journal of the Royal College of General Practitioners,* Occasional Paper 33.
Kapnio L A (1979), *Primary Health Care in Europe*. EURO Reports and Studies 14. Geneva: WHO.
Kempe C H, *et al.* (1962) The Battered Child Syndrome. *Journal of the American Medical Association,* **181**(1), pp. 7–14.
Körner E (1984), *Report of the Steering Group on Health Service Information Systems*. London: HMSO.
Lane K (1969), *The Longest Art*. London: George Allen & Unwin Ltd.
Loudon I S L (1985), *Medical Care and the General Practitioner 1750–1850*. Oxford: Clarendon Press.
Martin C (1987), Practice Makes Perfect? *Nursing Times,* **83**(17), pp. 28–31.
Mayston E (1969), *Report on the Management Structure in the Local Authority Nursing Services*. London: HMSO.
McEwan M (1959), *Health Visiting*. London: Faber and Faber.
National Health Service Act (1946), London: HMSO.
NHS and Community Care Act (1990), London: HMSO.
Nightingale F (1895), *Notes on Nursing: What it is and what it is not*. (Re-issued, 1974) London: Blackie.
Nuttall P D (1977), *Politics, Prejudices, Professionals: Nurses and Politics*. A paper presented to RCN Professional Conference, May 1977.
Ong B N, Humphris G, Annett H and Rifkin S. (1989), *Rapid Appraisal in an Urban Setting: An example from the developed world*. University of Keele.
Owen J (1978), Learning from each other. *Nursing Times, Community Option,* **Feb**, pp. 15–18.
Peachey M (1987), Practice Nurses A GP Employee? The Case For. *Nursing Times,* **83**(17), p 34.
Pereira Gray J (1982), The doctor's family: some problems and solutions. *Journal of the Royal College of General Practitioners,* **32**, pp. 75–79.
Reedy B L E, Philips P R, and Newell D J (1976), Nurses and Nursing in Primary Medical Care in England. *British Medical Journal,* **2**, pp. 1304–1306.
Royal College of General Practitioners (1981), *Report of the Working Party on Health and Prevention in Primary Care*. Report for General Practice 18. RCGP.
Royal College of Nursing (1977), Evidence to the Royal Commision on the National Health Service. London: RCN.

Royal College of Nursing (1984), *Report of a Working Party on Practice Nurse Training*. London: RCN.

Royal Commission (1972), *Reorganisation of Local Government Boundaries* (chaired by Lord Maud). London: HMSO.

Secretary of State for Social Services (1987), *Promoting Better Health: Government's Programme for Improving Primary Health Care*. London: HMSO.

Seebohm F (1968), *Report of the Local Authority and Allied Social Services Committee*. London: HMSO.

Shakespeare A (1989), I*nterprofessional Education in Primary Health Care. A National Survey*. London: CAIPE.

Stern W M (1966), *Britain Yesterday and Today: An Outline of Economic History from the middle of the Eighteenth Century*. Oxford: John Bellows.

Stilwell B (1985), Prevention and Health: the Concern of Nursing. *Journal of the Royal Society of Health,* **1,** pp. 31–34.

Stilwell B and Drury M (1988), Description and Evaluation of a course for practice nurses. *Journal of the Royal College of General Practitioners,* **38**, pp. 203–206.

Stilwell B and Hobbs R (eds) (1990), *Nursing in General Practice: Clinical Care Book 1*. Oxford: Radcliffe Medical Press.

Stocks M (1960), *A Hundred Years of District Nursing*. London: Allen and Unwin.

Travelbee J (1971), *Interpersonal Aspects of Nursing*. Philadelphia: J A Davis Co.

UKCC (1986), *Report of the Working Group: Project 2000. A New Preparation for Practice*. London: UKCC.

UKCC (1990), *Statement on Practice Nurses and Aspects of the New GP Contract*. London: UKCC.

UKCC (1991), *Consultative Document on the Future Practice and Education of Community Health Nurses*. London: UKCC.

UKCC (1992), *Code of Professional Conduct for the Nurse, Midwife and Health Visitor, 3rd edn*. London: UKCC.

WHO (1978), *Health for All: European Targets for Health*. Geneva: WHO.

WHICH? (1987), Making Your Doctor Better. *WHICH?,* **May 1987,** pp. 230–233.

Williams J (1979), Adult Education and Interprofessional Teaching. In England H, Education for Co-operation in Health and Social Work. *Journal of the Royal College of General Practitioners*. Occasional Paper 14, pp. 10–11.

2 Patient-centred decision making and clinical reasoning

Patient-centred clinical reasoning is central to all professional practice. In Chapter 1 an excerpt from the Griffiths report was cited charging nurses with a responsibility to exercise clinical judgement in the best interests of the patient. Chapter 1 discussed the development from practice nursing to nursing in general practice as a process of professional evolution. **Figure 1.3** described processes underpinning practice nursing. Problem solving and decision making processes are central if nurses are to progress and become autonomous professionals in the Primary Health Care Team.

In this chapter it is intended to consider what we understand by clinical reasoning, clinical judgement, problem solving and decision making in nursing and how this relates to assessment and treatment decisions taken. Initially, the importance of the area is considered and the types of problems that nurses solve and the decisions they make in general practice will be discussed. This will be followed by consideration of what is known about how people reason and the principles involved. The role of the patient and issues of communication will be discussed in relation to partnership between nurse and patient. The nature of expertise will be explored and the constraints and complex situations characteristic of general practice discussed. Finally, the question of how clinical judgement can be improved and implications for education will be addressed.

2.1 The importance of clinical reasoning

A central value of nursing is that it is a practice-based discipline. Further, the importance of primary health care has been highlighted by the World Health Organisation as the first point of contact in health services. In Chapter 1 the understanding of primary health care by the Royal College of General Practitioners was stated. This was a commitment to prevention and early detection or screening for vulnerability and presymptomatic disease and related health education. Nurses in general practice are centrally involved in these activities. As such, the ability to make judgements about patient groups who may be vulnerable to developing a particular problem is critical. Practice nurses are increasingly becoming the first point of contact for patients, although this represents a relatively small proportion of the primary contact within the practice. However, nurses need to be aware of some of the risks and side effects of first contact and need to be able to make an accurate assessment about status prior to intervention or appropriate referral. This implies both knowledge and skills at an advanced level. Nurses are engaged in screening for hypertension, cervical cytology, diabetes and asthma and many are directly in touch with the patients in the practice. However, they are also involved with secondary and tertiary intervention, for example post-operative care and the removal of sutures as well as chronic disability as indicated above, i.e. asthma, hypertension and diabetes.

The historical development of nursing in general practice was discussed in Chapter 1 charting the evolution of an increasingly autonomous profession. Why look at clinical reasoning? The clinical reasoning process can be suggested to be a problem-solving process leading to decisions about categorisation or diagnosis of nursing problems and the selection of treatment. An understanding of how reasoning can be improved or enhanced is important for developing professional practice and an autonomous professional.

The government White Paper 'Caring for People' (1990) suggests that professional practice and clinical decision making should be based on systematic assessment. The practice nurse is in a position to assess patient need systematically. What type of problem is encountered within the general practice setting? Acute health problems, the treatment of chronic lesions and advising about and administering immunisations are all examples of the surgery workload. All require a systematic assessment on the part of the nurse. For example, a patient may present with a lesion on the leg having been referred by the doctor for treatment. The doctor may have made a diagnosis, venous ulcer, and may have made recommendations concerning treatment. However, the nurse will assess pedal pulses to identify the quality of the circulation to the extremities. The nurse will assess the extent of the ulcerated area in considering how the patient's leg will be dressed and will question the patient about susceptibility to allergic reactions and the success of previous interventions if this is a recurrence.

The nurse may also take the opportunity to explore the patient's level of physical activity, the amount of time spent standing still and the position of the legs whilst sitting: all factors known to influence venous return. Social considerations such as the nature of the patient's job may also influence the choice of treatment.

This patient could return to the nurse for several weeks for redressing. On one of these occasions the nurse observes that the patient looks more frail, pale and sad than usual. When questioned it transpires that a very close friend with whom she had been at school has recently died; the patient is now the only member of a small circle of friends dating from those days still alive. This patient is a single woman living alone. The nurse will decide the course of action based on an assessment of psychological status. This may take the form of an appropriate referral or a supportive nursing intervention, making professional colleagues aware of the patient's loss. Whatever decision is made about the course of action to be taken it should follow a systematic psychological and social assessment on the part of the nurse resulting in a clinical decision. Anecdotal evidence suggests that this is not always the case.

The ability to assess is central to nursing practice in order to function effectively within the primary health care team. Increasingly patients self-refer for apparently 'minor' ailments, conditions they describe as trivial, not wishing to trouble the doctor. If the nurse is the primary contact it is likely that a range of patient problems that may or may not be the presenting problem will be encountered. For example a mother brings her child into the surgery complaining that the child has a small scald that is painful. As part of the nursing assessment it is noted that the mother is tense and distracted and the child quiet and apparently 'well behaved'. When examining the child bruises are present on both arms and trunk, and the mother is a little unclear about how they were sustained. The nurse knows that childrens' limbs are frequently bruised but is surprised by the bruising to the trunk. Whilst chatting to the mother, in an apparently informal fashion, the nurse learns that her partner has gone to live with someone else. As a consequence the woman is distressed and money is very tight, she has been taking in typing at home in an attempt to cope. The nurse has considered the wellbeing of both mother and child and based on her assessment judges that the appropriate course of action is referral. She suspects a potential problem in the relationship between mother and child and that the initial contact was a cry for help. It may not be a direct nursing intervention that is needed, but a clear nursing assessment resulting in a possible diagnosis, in this case, the risk of child abuse and a parent experiencing acute psychological problems due to life events and life stresses. The nursing intervention is appropriate referral. The nature of the referral will be laid down by local policy to which the nurse must adhere rather than take independent action for which she is not prepared.

The North American Nurses Association defines a nursing diagnosis as follows:

> A nursing diagnosis is a clinical judgement about individual, family or community responses to actual or potential health problems/life processes. Nursing diagnoses provide the basis for selection of nursing interventions to achieve outcomes for which the nurse is accountable. (Carroll-Johnson, 1990, p 50).

The American Nurses Association (1980) suggests that 'nursing is the diagnosis and treatment of human responses to actual or potential health problems'. There are problems with such a definition in that it is not exclusive to nursing (Miers, 1991). However, the emphasis on assessment prior to planning and intervention is essential. Much of the work concerning clinical reasoning and the nature of nursing problems emanates from North America; for this reason American definitions are cited in this text. Practice nurses do need to diagnose in order to refer as well as treat directly. They have frequent contact with practice patients and can be suggested to have a pivotal position in the primary health care team. It is now intended to consider how people solve problems and make decisions.

2.2 Problem solving and decision making

The processes of problem solving and decision making will be discussed in relation to psychological research, research into doctor's reasoning processes and research with nurses. It is suggested that all are relevant because it is the processes that are of interest and these processes are common to human reasoning, although they may vary according to the nature of the problem.

Problem solving in medicine has been described as a process of making adequate decisions based on inadequate information (Elstein *et al.*, 1978). Problem solving has been suggested to be behaviour that is organised toward some goal (Anderson, 1985). Three essential features of problem solving are goal directedness, identification of subgoals or interim stages and the selection of the means to achieve the goal (Padrick, 1990). Making a decision has been treated as making a choice between alternatives (Slovic *et al.*, 1977). Decisions are made during the process of problem solving (Elstein *et al.*, 1978; McWhinney, 1972).

Considerable research has been carried out into the processes involved when people solve problems and make decisions, although the area of study is by its nature complex. Much of the applied research has been conducted with doctor's diagnostic decisions because of the perceived importance of these decisions and the cost of error. Different approaches have been adopted in the area as a whole. The early work with medical decisions worked within a model of rational behaviour; human decisions were compared with those that would be predicted by a mathematical model based on probability theory using the same information (Slovic *et al.*, 1977). There has also been concern regarding the total problem solving process and how we process information in order to solve problems (Newell and Simon, 1972). More recent research with nurses has taken a slightly different approach, focusing on reasoning during the course of and as a result of action (Benner, 1984). But prior to considering the cognitive processes it may be useful to consider the social situations in which clinical decisions are made and some of the factors that influence them.

2.3 Factors influencing assessment and reasoning

Professional judgements can be influenced by many factors such as beliefs, values and personal preferences. Stockwell (1975) noted that some patients appeared to be avoided by nurses. She conducted a small study directly observing nurse–patient interactions. Those patients who received the least nursing attention were older and complained more, they gave less positive feedback. Although patients cannot be avoided in general practice, some can receive more attention than others. The situational nature of clinical decision making has been observed with doctors (Stein, 1991). For some doctors the overall objective was the satisfaction of the patient with the decision made, rather than being solely concerned with the medical rigour. Personal circumstances were also found to influence the course of action taken. An example was cited of a married couple with a small child, both of whom were doctors. When the female partner was working at night the husband's clinical evaluation of a telephone call at 2 a.m. from a nurse requesting his presence at a nursing home was influenced by considerations of their child's care. Another influence observed was the day of the week where short cuts were taken in order to get away for the weekend (Stein, 1991).

Fondiller, Rosage and Neuhaus (1990) described patient-centred values amongst occupational therapists that influenced their approach to treatment. The therapists sampled expressed values that emphasised a therapeutic relationship, taking sufficient time to take a complete history and the treatment of the whole person. These values may be directly at odds with a climate of cost containment and short hospital stays but arguably may actually be associated with effective intervention. This was a small study involving 12 therapists only, but it is of interest in the current context. We do not make judgements in a vacuum. Pressures such as economic factors and pressure to deal with large numbers of people in a finite amount of time can influence both the assessment and its scope and consequent intervention decisions. The management of time will be discussed at a later point but the priority given to the clinical reasoning process may well substantially affect the outcome for the patient.

2.4 Clinical reasoning

Studies of the diagnostic reasoning processes of nurses and doctors describe a similar sequence of steps (Elstein *et al.*, 1978; Tanner, 1989). When making an initial assessment both nurses and doctors generated hypotheses about possible diagnoses or patient problems, such as the presence of infection, based on presenting signs and symptoms and their overall impression of the patient. They were doing two things. They were using both verbal and non-verbal information to form an overall impression of the patient and using that impression to formulate possible ideas about patient status at the beginning of the assessment process. They then used those ideas to guide their search for further information. They searched for and collected information that would either confirm or refute these diagnostic hypotheses. The ideas or hypotheses were guiding the search and making the reasoning process manageable. An evaluation was then made in order to either determine a diagnosis or determine whether it was necessary to start the process again. The theoretical approach being taken was a problem solving or information processing approach.

From the vast literature that addresses clinical problem solving and judgement certain principles have been established. Clinical problems are very broad and open, unlike problems such as catching a train from a particular station. The end point, the station, is known; the task is to work out how to get there. Clinical problems need to be made manageable. Take, for example, judging the current health status of a patient. This is a huge problem and is made manageable by converting it from a large open problem with an infinite number of possibilities to a more circumscribed problem (Weinman, 1981). The evidence suggests that the patient's presenting signs and symptoms, overall appearance and the impression that is made assist in this process. Recall the mother and child. The nurse generates a possible patient problem or diagnosis based on the overall impression that is made, both verbal and non-verbal cues. The tentative diagnosis can then serve to limit the search for further information to support it or otherwise. The strategy makes the task manageable; we know there are limits to what we can attend to at any one time (Kahneman, 1973). Personal experience suggests that we can only attend to a limited number of environmental events simultaneously. Should the first attempt to solve the problem be fruitless, the human problem solver starts the process again.

This approach does run counter to what was thought to be the tradition of taking a full history before making any inferences. However, jumping to conclusions based on preconceived expectations and incomplete information and knowledge, premature foreclosure, is worthy of extreme caution. The process may be as rapid or as time-consuming as the complexity of the situation and the expertise of the professional determine. A critical point in the process is the testing of an idea or hypothesis to fit with the information available. A further observation is that people are not very good at looking for information that will show that their ideas are incorrect; they tend to look for information as confirmation (Wason, 1966; Kahneman and Tversky, 1973). Elstein *et al.* (1978) characterised medical decisions as the making of adequate decisions with inadequate information but recognising the significance of the information. All the possible alternatives and the relevant statistical information may not be available and as a consequence errors will occur periodically. What we set out to do is minimise error. In order to use information it has to be available and its significance understood. Where doctors realised the significance of statistical information about base rates of certain diseases, they used that information in their reasoning (Christiansen-Szalanski and Bushyhead, 1981).

The implication for nursing in general practice is in terms of concern for both the adequacy of the knowledge base and insight into limitations and influences on the clinical reasoning process resulting in professional decision making. This insight is useful in general practice where complex decisions are made such as the administration of vaccine. The use of a protocol in the form of a decision tree or flow chart can facilitate the decision process as illustrated in **Figure 2.1**.

A flow chart can hinder the decision process if nurses follow it too rigidly. It is an aid to decision making, ensuring a minimum standard, not the decision process itself.

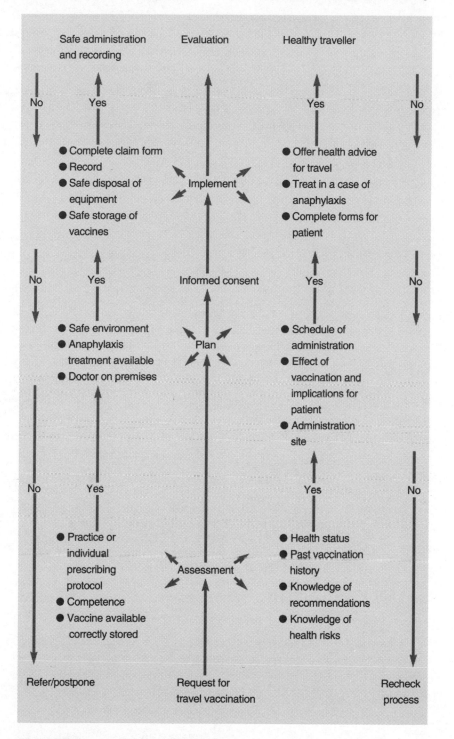

Figure 2.1 Flow chart for travel vaccinations.

2.5 Rapid judgements

The preceding discussion has been concerned with a problem solving approach; however, nurses make assessments and judgements very rapidly during the course of practice. Rapid intuitive assessments made by nurses during the course of practice have been studied (Benner, 1984). The strategies of experienced and less experienced nurses were described. It was observed that the experienced nurses made very rapid accurate decisions, apparently recognising critical verbal and non-verbal cues and ignoring the irrelevant. The expert nurses appeared to know certain inter-relationships between cues that are critical and be able to predict particular patient states and responses, hence their ability to attend to the information they judged to be relevant and to ignore the irrelevant. A further study of very experienced nurses working in critical or intensive care suggested that the nurses made deliberate assessments and made rapid intuitive judgements dependent upon the circumstances (Etheredge, 1989).

An experienced nurse may recognise critical cues and the relationship between these cues but less experienced colleagues may have to pursue a more lengthy process of assessment. Further, they may overlook cues that the experienced nurse detects, such as psychological cues in response to a procedure that indicate an underlying anxiety about health. An inexperienced nurse may also become side-tracked by irrelevant information and overlook what is relevant, hence take longer to recognise relationships between the cues observed. As a consequence, intervention may be a staged process rather than being directed at the central issues. For example, a patient presents for a blood test prior to surgery. An experienced nurse notes that the bleeding time following venepuncture appears prolonged and alerts colleagues. A less experienced nurse may not be alert in the first instance to the significance of this sign and may pay more attention to the patient's anxiety prior to surgery. Benner further noted that very experienced nurses recognised a patient problem without necessarily being able to justify their reason in scientific terms. They had a hunch and recognised cues they had met before without being able to put their finger on anything really tangible.

The above work can again be set in the context of expectation. Assessments were made about the affective status of hospital inpatients by student nurses at different stages of training. The assessments of those at the beginning of training were shown to be influenced by how they judged they would feel in the same position as the patient. However, the assessments of the third year students were more similar to judgements they made about a typical patient in that position (Openshaw, 1984). The nurses appeared to be using a rule of thumb to help them to make the assessment and expectations developed with experience.

In summary, it is the situation and the nature of the problem that appears to determine the strategies that people employ during the course of clinical reasoning. Personal knowledge, values, beliefs and circumstances also affect how the decision goal is perceived as well as the verbal and non-verbal signals given by the patient.

2.6 The role of the patient in decision making

In the previous section the patient was barely mentioned, the emphasis of the research briefly described was on reasoning processes and strategies. It is now intended to turn to issues of patient-centred decision making, a value shared by many different professional groups. If a nurse is making a diagnosis about a particular patient, for example, that they are overweight, the decision problem then becomes how the nurse can intervene most effectively and help the patient to lose weight. Central to the effectiveness of the intervention is the cooperation of the patient and a willingness to modify behaviour. The implication is that the patient perceives that there is a problem also and is, indeed, willing to take advice in order to achieve the intended goal, target weight. There may be a need for the nurse and patient to form what has been termed a therapeutic alliance (Madden, 1990). Many people may seek help in order to lose weight, because they are self motivated in the first instance and wish to find an effective vehicle for achieving their goal. However, where the nurse diagnoses a problem, in order for any change to take place the patient also needs to share and accept that diagnosis.

Madden (1990) distinguished between therapeutic alliance and compliance. In compliance the patient is persuaded to co-operate with the treatment, whereas with therapeutic alliance the patient becomes a client involved in the negotiation with the nurse, both parties being allies in achieving a common goal. The implication is a partnership between nurse and client rather than an authoritarian stance, however socially skilled, on the part of the professional. The nurse has professional knowledge that is useful to the partnership, the patient has personal knowledge about life style, beliefs, values and attitudes. The nurse may need to work within the patient's reality, for example, achieving a target weight that is acceptable to that patient. A person from a cultural background where the family meal is a central focus and sexual attraction is associated with a 'well-covered' body, a target weight may not be that prescribed by the norms. However, both may be working toward a goal of developing health behaviours that are consistent with the patient's health status and lifestyle through a process of negotiation.

It may be useful to consider the above issues in relation to health screening taking place in all practices. There is an implicit directive within policy that has instigated much of the screening toward assessing individuality rather than recognising the person as part of a social unit. Take the new patient check and a new 16-year-old patient found to be overweight. The nurse may wish to go beyond the individual and work with the family on dietary advice.

Research has been carried out to identify the reasons for dissatisfaction amongst patients and has found it to be linked to the quality of the relationship between professional and patient. A study attempting to identify the reasons for dissatisfaction and insecurity amongst patients in Finland has been carried out with two groups totalling three hundred and forty patients. It was found that the quality of the relationship between carer and patient predicted most of the variance associated with dissatisfaction (Raatikainen, 1991). Dissatisfaction and reports of insecurity were significantly correlated ($r = 0.63$ and $r = 0.53$, $p < 0.001$). Patients appreciated and felt safe with care that they felt was well planned and goal oriented.

Allowing patients to be actively involved by encouraging them to ask questions has also been associated with reports of satisfaction (Greenfield *et al.*, 1985). Further work suggests a gender difference in the willingness of patients to ask questions spontaneously (Weisman and Teitelbaum, 1989). Women were found to ask more questions; men talked more and were more likely to interrupt. The interpretation of these observations may not be straightforward, as there will be individual differences in assertiveness, desire to be involved as well as gender differences in communication patterns. However, these are useful observations and it is worth 'checking out' whether a patient would like to be better informed or more involved. When nurses offered terminally ill patients control in terms of choice or decision making opportunities they almost always took it (Pepler and Lynch, 1991). A review of the literature about doctor–patient communication, estimated from the studies reviewed that doctors talked for about 60% of the time and patients 40% (Roter *et al.*, 1988). A further observation when considering the amount of information given to patients was that black patients received less information than any other group. The opportunity for patient-centred decision making must have been reduced for this group.

2.7 Constraints of practice

Constraints of practice that are common across different settings are the constraints of time and opportunity, albeit to different degrees. Characteristic of general practice is the large number of patients being seen within a prescribed time frame. It is under conditions of time pressure where it is critical to make the maximum use of opportunities, because unlike the hospital setting the patient leaves the surgery. As a result, they are not available for re-assessments and further intervention. In hospital, staff can return to the patient at a later point and have the opportunity for re-evaluating patient status. Skilled performance in general practice that reflects a clear understanding of the times when it is necessary to make an assessment that goes beyond the initial patient report is likely to make the most of opportunity available. Skilled performance would view the patient within their social context and consider psychological and physical factors. This does imply the considerable expertise inherent in nursing in general practice.

A further potential constraint is that of ownership versus autonomy, that is of the nurse as an independent decision maker with a specific body of knowledge rather than solely following instruction. This does imply educational preparation for the role at an advanced level. A major impediment to clinical reasoning is that the clinical competencies that characterise nursing in general practice are currently ill defined (Damant, 1990). Competence can be viewed as a psychological construct with elements of knowledge, skill and values. Clinical reasoning uses knowledge to select skills, and values underpin the total process. An example of competence could be illustrated when undertaking venepuncture. A male patient is sent by the doctor for a non-routine blood test. The nurse notes that the patient is asthmatic and further notes that he has not requested a repeat prescription during the last 3 months.

The patient is prescribed Becotide for prophylactic control of his asthma. The nurse questions the patient about how he is feeling and is told that he is feeling so much better that he has decided that he no longer needs his medication. The nurse takes this opportunity to explain the reasons for the medication, reinforcing previous explanations. Together, they arrive at the decision to recommence his medication and monitor his peak flow readings.

The competency demonstrated by the nurse was the use of knowledge of the patient's medical condition and its likely course to predict a possible health outcome. An apparent lack of compliance with treatment instructions was identified using skills of observation and questioning. Explanatory and negotiating skills resulted in the patient's decision to recommence his medication and monitor his progress. The nurse's values suggest to her that the patient should have maximum control over his condition. She appreciated that he may not have fully understood and accepted his condition, indeed the explanation may have been perfunctory. The nurse achieved a therapeutic alliance with this patient.

Further potential constraints that may be imposed by social policy and the contract could be in terms of a numbers game or pay game focusing purely on tasks at the level of the individual. Both tasks and people are important, but the nursing focus can be suggested to be on the individual person within their own social unit. The emphasis on assessment within recent social policy does emphasise its importance.

2.8 Expertise and experience

From the preceding discussion it is evident that expertise implies a clear understanding of role and function. That is an understanding of the nature of the problems to be solved. A critical component of problem solving is to understand the nature of the problem. In this context, it means the full implications of the nurse's role for a particular patient. Such an understanding suggests considerable thought about the scope of nursing with the necessary knowledge, skills and values. This implies education and preparation for that role as well as experience.

Expert nurses have been shown to make very rapid assessments and decisions, recognising critical signs and symptoms, ignoring irrelevance and using the impression that they have formed to lead them to further information. They are able to predict the likely outcomes from difference courses of action and using their knowledge select an action. Rapid and accurate assessment made by very experienced nurses may be characterised by a clear understanding of the nature and structure of a situation and a rapid recognition of relevant cues that relate to a patient state. This is a very rapid process of problem solving. **Table 2.1** suggests differences that may distinguish between different levels of expertise. Three levels are suggested: experienced nurses, nurses with advanced skills and nurses with autonomous expertise. For nursing in general practice to develop the nursing role the level of expertise needs to be set at an appropriate level.

Table 2.1 Clinical reasoning expertise.

Experienced	*Advanced*	*Expertise*
General knowledge General skills Appreciates research findings	More knowledge Developed skills Some research skills	Focused depth of knowledge Focused and fully developed skills Research ability advancing the practice of others
Assimilation of information and selection of appropriate courses of action	Rapid assimilation of information and recognition of a range of alternative actions	Rapid assimilation of information and recognition of critical cues. Recognition of a full range of alternative actions
Anticipates and evaluates outcome from chosen course of action	Anticipates and speculates on the outcomes from different courses of action	Predicts outcomes from different courses of action with increased accuracy

Table 2.1 illustrates increasing reasoning skills that are coupled with a depth of professional knowledge and clinical skill. There is an increasing ability to make the most of a practice situation. How can autonomous expertise be developed amongst less experienced nurses in general practice?

2.9 Developing practice

Benner would imply that practice is a major factor. However, practice or experience per se may be insufficient in a complex situation. The performance of third year student nurses diagnosing post-operative complications was observed to improve as a result of practice with making such diagnoses (Openshaw, 1984). Elstein *et al.* (1978) found that practice with relevant clinical tasks resulted in improved performance, that is practice solving relevant problems. One of the implications for professional development within a busy practice is to seek out problems to solve and compare the outcome with an expert colleague.

A slightly different approach is illustrated in Benner's work and has been described as reflective practice (Schon, 1983). It relates to action carried out as a result of assessment. The nurse asks questions about critical incidents in the surgery, that is incidents where things went very well or when they appeared to be unsatisfactory. The implications for developing practice are firstly, to question what is being done but also again to enlist the support of a colleague with expertise. The nurse and colleague can explore together the characteristics that seemed to contribute to the good practice and consider what could have been done differently where there was dissatisfaction. Reflective practice is more than thoughtful practice: it requires that the professional constantly questions the actions that are taken and learns as a result of improvisation during the course of practice, identifying successful actions. There is evidence to suggest that we cannot teach people to solve problems directly. Rather, we can supply problems that will help to develop their problem-solving skills, that is problems of increasing complexity, and we can help them to reflect on that process. Further opportunities for continuing education need to be sought in order to develop expertise fully.

Practice can only develop fully if there is adequate recording, a data base to ensure continuity of care. The process of care needs to be recorded; this skill can be developed in conjunction with problem solving skills. Succinct record writing does require practice. Continuity and legality are major considerations and records should contain information about the assessment, interventions and decisions, any risk factors and precautions and criteria defined to evaluate outcome (see **Figure 2.1**). The Lloyd George documentation does impose constraints but the issue needs resolving in a consumer-oriented society because of issues of accountability and litigation. The growth of alternative forms of record keeping, information technology and computers in the practice will have the potential to revolutionise recording in the future.

Summary

Both the situation and the nature of the problem influence the strategies that are employed during clinical reasoning. Nurses use a variety of verbal and non-verbal signals given by patients. Understanding what is critical and the nature of the problem characterises expertise. However, the way in which decision goals are perceived is influenced by personal knowledge, values, beliefs and circumstances.

In conclusion, nurses in general practice work in a complex and pressured environment. The nurse is a general practitioner in her or his own right. Within the context of nursing practice she or he is able to select appropriate nursing interventions and refer for medical input or input from health and social care colleagues at an appropriate point. It is critical that nurses work within the bounds of their competence and seek education to assist with their professional development if nursing is to develop within general practice. Education for the future needs to address this issue.

References

American Nurses Association (1980), in Pinkley C L (1991) Exploring NANDA's Definition of Nursing Diagnosis: Linking Diagnostic Judgements with the Selection of Outcomes and Interventions. *Nursing Diagnosis* 2(1), pp. 26–32.

Anderson J R (1985), *Cognitive Psychology and its Implications.* New York: W H Freeman and Co.

Benner P (1984), *From Novice to Expert.* Menlo Park, California: Addison-Wesley Publishing Co.

Caring for People (1990), Government White Paper. London: HMSO.

Carroll-Johnson R M (1990), *Reflections on the Ninth Biennial Conference.* Nursing Diagnosis, 1, p. 50.

Christiansen-Szalanski J J J and Bushyhead J B (1981), Physicians' Use of Probabilistic Information in a Real Clinic Setting. *Journal of Experimental Psychology: Human Perception and Performance*, 7, pp. 928–935.

Damant M (1990), *Report of the Review Group for the Education and Training for Practice Nursing 'The Challenges of Primary Health Care in the 1990s'.* London: (ENB).

Elstein A S, Schulman L S, and Sprafka S A (1978), *Medical Problem Solving: an Analysis of Clinical Reasoning.* Cambridge, Massachusetts: Harvard University Press.

Etheridge C L O (1989), *An Analysis of Critical Care Nurses' Clinical Decision Making.* Unpublished Ed D Dissertation, University of San Francisco.

Fondiller E D, Rosage L J, and Neuhaus B E (1990), Values influencing clinical reasoning in occupational therapy: an exploratory study. *Occupational Therapy Journal of Research*, 10, pp. 41–45.

Greenfield S, Kaplan S, and Ware J E (1985), Expanding Patient Involvement in Care. Effects on Patient Outcomes. *Annual International Medicine,* 102, pp. 520–528.

Kahneman D (1973), *Attention and Effort.* Englewood Cliffs, New Jersey: Prentice-Hall.

Kahneman D and Tversky A (1973), On the Psychology of Prediction. *Psychological Review,* 80, pp. 237–281.

Madden B P (1990), The Hybrid Model for Concept Development: its value for the study of therapeutic alliance. *Advances in Nursing Science*, **April**, pp. 75–87.

McWhinney I R (1972), Problem Solving and Decision Making in Primary Medical Practice. *Proceedings of the Royal Society of Medicine*, 65, pp. 934–938.

Miers L J (1991), NANDA's Definition of Nursing Diagnosis: a plea for conceptual clarity. *Nursing Diagnosis*, 2, pp. 9–18.

Newell A and Simon H A (1972), *Human Problem Solving.* Englewood Cliffs, New Jersey: Prentice-Hall.

Openshaw S (1984), *Clinical Judgements by Nurses: Decision Strategies and Nurses' Appraisal of Patient Affect.* Unpublished PhD Dissertation, University of London.

Padrick K P (1990), *Clinical Decision Making in Nursing. A Comparison of Simulations and Practice Situations.* Unpublished PhD Dissertation, Oregon Health Sciences University.

Pepler C J and Lynch A (1991), Relational messages of control in nurse–patient interactions with terminally ill patients with AIDS and cancer. *Journal of Palliative Care,* 7, 18–29.

Raatikainen R (1991), Dissatisfaction and Insecurity of Patients in Domiciliary Care. *Journal of Advanced Nursing,* 16, pp. 154–164.

Roter D L, Hall J A, and Katz N R (1988), Patient–Physician Communication: A Descriptive Summary of the Literature. Patient Education and Counselling, 12, pp. 99–119.

Schon D A (1983), *The Reflective Practitioner.* New York: Basic Books Inc.

Slovic P, Fischoff B and Lichtenstein S (1977), Behavioural Decision Theory. *Annual Review of Psychology,* **28**, pp. 1–39.

Stein H F (1991), The Role of Some Nonbiomedical Parameters in Clinical Decision Making: an Ethnographic Approach. *Qualitative Health Research,* **1**, pp. 6–26.

Stockwell F (1975), *The Unpopular Patient. The Study of Nursing Care.* London: Royal College of Nursing.

Tanner C A (1989), Use of Research in Clinical Judgement. In C A Lindeman and C A Tanner (eds) *Using Nursing Research.* New York: National League for Nursing.

Wason P C (1966), Reasoning. In B M Foss (ed) *New Horizons in Psychology.* Harmondsworth, England: Penguin.

Weinman J (1981), *An Outline of Psychology as Applied to Medicine.* Bristol: John Wright.

Weisman C S and Teitelbaum M A (1989), Women and Health Care Communication. *Patient Education and Counselling,* **13**, pp. 183–199.

3 Developing the framework for clinical practice

The previous chapter has emphasised the role of clinical reasoning and its importance in decision making for the nurse in general practice. This decision making takes place within a complex and pressurised environment in terms of limitations of consultation time, the potential health needs of the patient and the colleague/employee relationship with the GP. This chapter encourages nurses to reflect on their position within the practice both in the context of the delivery of clinical care and their interprofessional relationship with the GP. It offers an opportunity for reflection on a framework for delivery of care and on which to develop clinical reasoning.

Nursing has been able to become a potential change agent within general practice mainly because of the lack of hierarchal and autocratic management structure typical of some organisations. The experience of bureaucracy goes some way to explain why nurses in general practice defended their right to remain employed by general practitioners in spite of the recommendations made in the Community Nursing Review (Cumberlege, 1986). The professional and employment relationship between the nurse and the GP cannot be underestimated and has done much to contribute to the development of nursing and meeting the health needs of the practice population. The GP, the employer of the nurse, has the contractual responsibility for the patients registered with him but the nurse remains professionally accountable for the care she herself gives to the patient. It is also clearly laid down in the '*Red Book*' (Statement of Fees and Allowances payable to General Medical Practitioners) that it is expected that nurses are to hold the qualifications of and have regard to the 'appropriate national regulatory body' (DOH, 1990).

However, nursing in general practice raises criticism from the nursing profession because of its relative dependence within a medically dominated environment. In specifically relating to items of service for which the GP receives target payments (immunisation, vaccination and cytology) it is also stated that these items may be claimed for by him even if provided by staff working 'at his or her direction'. It is this vicarious responsibility that gives rise to issues of professional accountability, dependence and independence within the employer/employee relationship.

3.1 Approaches to care

The underlying framework for nursing practice is the assessment, planning, implementation and evaluation of patient care. The principles on which this framework is based are dependent on the overall perspective of care and the clinical reasoning behind that perspective. The traditional nursing approach has been based on a procedural framework which emphasises the nurse's role as one that alleviates symptoms and mediates medical treatment in relation to pathology and medical diagnoses. An example of this approach is illustrated for the care of the non-insulin-dependent diabetic patient (**Table 3.1**).

Clearly, nursing does mediate medical treatment and helps patients to cope with problems arising from disease processes. However, as the nursing profession seeks to emphasise nursing as a specific discipline, the emphasis moves more to assisting the person in their daily living activities in spite of whatever problems arise through disability or disease. Areas of care may include increasing the person's self knowledge and their independence within the context of their need and/or environment. This different emphasis is again illustrated for the care of the non-insulin-dependent diabetic patient (**Table 3.2**).A comparison in more general terms is suggested in **Table 3.3**.

Table 3.1 A procedural framework based on tasks for care for the non-insulin-dependent diabetic patient.

DOCTOR
diagnoses diabetes

NURSE

Assessment	Planning	Implementation	Evaluation
CARRIES out tasks delegated by doctor: e.g. venepuncture urinalysis visual acuity checks feet dietary advice May include: psychological and social assessment	Explains and arranges tests with patient	Performs tasks	Tasks performed
			DOCTOR informed

Table 3.2 Framework for care of the non-insulin-dependent diabetic patient based on a nursing model.

<u>DOCTOR</u>
diagnoses diabetes

<u>NURSE</u>

Assessment	Planning	Implementation	Evaluation
<u>ASSESS</u> with patient problems/potential problems with: nutrition eye sight mobility urinary function, etc.	Identifies areas needing care, e.g. nutrition Talks and plans approach with patient (and relatives) Arranges tests, e.g. venepuncture	Intervention according to need which may include **Tests:** venepuncture urinalysis blood pressure **Advice:** re diet **Education:** teaching self care	1) Avoidance of potential problems 2) Self care by patient in relation to urinalysis 3) Increase of patient's know-ledge in relation to, e.g. diet
Psychological: acceptance of disease **Social**: family, etc. environment			
			<u>DOCTOR</u> informed of results and nursing history discussed

---

Table 3.3 Differences in nursing practice.

Nursing process	Traditional nursing (medical)
The nurse acts autonomously. The doctor is regarded as a colleague. Independent function	Deference to medicine and to the doctor. Dependent function
Nursing is an intellectual activity. The nurse is a creative thinker. Thus emphasis on intellectual skills	Nursing is a practical activity. The nurse performs. Thus emphasis on technical skills
The nurse actively seeks information	The nurse passively receives information
Work is dynamic	Work is routinised
Work is patient centred	Work is task centred
The nurse's role is expanded to the behavioural and social sciences	Nurse's role is restricted to physical aspects
The nurse is involved with the patient	The nurse avoids involvement with the patient as mechnanism against anxiety

Table 3.3 Differences in nursing practice *cont.*

Nursing process	Traditional nursing (medical)
The patient is an active participant	The patient is a passive receiver
The nurse is accountable for her actions individually	Accountability is diffused among the staff and delegated to a hierarchy
Ends-assessment	Means-assessment

Adapted from De la Cuesta (1979)

3.1.1 Procedural framework

Although a distinct nursing perspective has emerged, this remains an uncertain and indistinct concept for many colleagues, both nursing and medical, as well as for patients.

There is a suggestion that other disciplines regard nursing as an extension of their own professional group because they themselves are trained to diagnose using a pathophysiologic model (Carnevali *et al.*, 1984). For the nurse in general practice this perception is possibly increased because nursing intervention within the surgery/health centre is more technically based in comparison with her district nurse colleagues; the district nurse's role is perceived to be with the 'sick' and therefore associated with a more 'caring' role. In interviews with 153 nurses (both GP and health authority employed) in 113 practices which included rural and urban areas, 43 activities carried out by nurses were classified as:

● *'Caring'* activities, e.g. bed baths.
● *'Intermediate'* activities for which nurses and doctors are trained, e.g. blood pressure measurement.
● *'Technical'* activities, e.g. immunisations (Reedy *et al.*, 1980).

Nursing in general practice can therefore be easily related to a procedural framework for care, the GP using the skills of the nurse as an assistant and technician. The nursing role appears to become more 'medicalised' and that may lead to professional dilemmas.

This framework also lends itself to the contractual relationship which the nurse in general practice holds to the employing GP. As such, she is required as part of that professional relationship to carry out certain medically oriented activities. There can be a degree of professional disquiet at being asked to undertake certain work and this leads on to the issue as to how these differences are expressed and handled within the team. There are some indications that this contractual relationship, which for all nurses has some relevance, only succeeds when:

> the nurse and doctor are both satisfied that the medical prescriptions and nursing actions are in the best interests of the patients: and where there are differences there is mutual professional effort to understand and resolve the different professional perspectives and to agree on the most suitable compromise

(Pembrey, 1984).

This does happen most of the time. However, if the nurse in general practice is to develop a role as a practitioner of nursing, become autonomous and be accountable for her care within the code of conduct for her profession, it seems more appropriate for her to work within the framework of nursing. Procedures then are carried out within a framework of holistic care and are not an isolated '**task**'.

The complementary roles of nursing and medicine are such that although they are distinct by the nature of the preparation, skills and knowledge, they overlap in promoting health. The doctor has a greater role in diagnosing and treating a disease process. The nurse has a greater role in maximising the patient's lifestyle in spite of a medical diagnosis (McFarlane and Castledine, 1982).

It must be stated that, while the medical role in 1982 was perceived to be tending towards the pragmatic approach, general practice in particular has re-evaluated its terms of reference. This has already been discussed in Chapter 1, and the increased concern with promotion of health and the limiting of disability has been described. This re-evaluation is also reflected in the 1982 GP Vocational Act. The Regulations stipulated that a doctor wishing to be a principal in general medical practice could only be accepted if he or she could 'provide a Certificate of either prescribed or equivalent experience' or provide a statement giving the reasons for exemption. The Membership examination of the RCGP is based on the job definition defined by the RCGP (1972). These areas are:

- Clinical practice – health and disease.
- Clinical practice – human development.
- Clinical practice – human behaviour.
- Medicine and society.
- The practice.

3.1.2 Nursing framework

Using a nursing framework reminds the nurse in general practice to develop a knowledge base and gives a secure foundation for practice. It may also identify for the GP and other colleagues the potential scope for nursing skills. In the early 1980s many nurses employed by GPs were spending much of their time in clerical and reception duties, and this could be considered as a poor use of resources (Gambrill, 1980). Conversely, however, in an earlier study, it was suggested that nursing abilities were highly valued at the initial contact for patients coming into the practice. This first impression was probably the most important function within any practice (Reedy, 1972). A significant minority of nurses still appear to be involved with clerical and reception duties. A profile of practice nurses in the South East Thames Region indicates 8% are carrying out reception work — 25% of these in rural practices (Warrier, 1992). While this may be appropriate for the practice needs, it should also raise questions as to whether or not nursing skills are being effectively utilised.

Nursing tends to be perceived by others within the description of tasks, functions and activities. However, it is also about teaching, advocacy and clinical judgement and it is in describing these processes that the nursing framework can be promoted. It is the special quality of nursing and nurses to have 'the ability to blend knowledge, skill, experience and empathy into seemingly effortless clinical practice' (Clarke, 1992).

Nurses in general practice need to and do address the aim of their clinical care and then assess, plan and implement care towards that aim. Reference has already been made in Chapter 1 to developments in nursing which resulted in conceptual frameworks and further reading is widely available. However, in the context of this book, it is for nurses to ensure that they can identify the intended outcome of their care, whether it is self care, promoting adaptation for lifestyle, independence or informed health choices.

Different situations will warrant different outcomes and this is as much to do with the values and beliefs of the practitioner concerning health and society, and the environment, as with the nature of individual patients and their needs. This could mean selecting a specific framework from the literature or creating a framework unique to their particular setting.

It is a challenge and a dilemma for the nurse in general practice to select a framework appropriate for her and for the needs of the patients being treated. She needs to choose how far she is willing to develop autonomy and to take on the responsibility that is necessarily implied with that full autonomy. Much may depend on her professional background and experience. Within these challenges she may encounter the potential difficulties of being employed by another profession which may not be willing to facilitate this role.

3.2 Interprofessional relationships between the nurse and the GP

Debate between the employer and the nurse on professional issues could be an impediment to improving clinical practice. On the other hand it can be the stimulant for professional collaboration and recognition of shared and individual skills. Evidence of tensions in the expectations of nursing in general practice emerged from the consultation process that resulted in the review of practice nursing (Damant, 1990). One message was that much existing practice is '**task**' based and procedure oriented. However, the second message that emerged was that there is a danger of presenting a practice profile that undermines the level of expertise involved.

The expertise involved is demonstrated in the examples of patient care given in the last chapter, where potential and actual problems are recognised over and above the initial reason for the consultation. It is therefore essential that the nurse is able to demonstrate her framework of care explicitly in the documentation of patient care. This will not only offer written evidence of the nursing perspective but will also assist in evaluating standards for care.

It may be possible for the nurse and GP to be in disagreement over a prescription for care or the necessity of a procedure. However, clinical reasoning based on sound knowledge skills and values offer the nurse confidence in discussing the matter and resolving it on an interprofessional basis. For example:

- The GP may direct the nurse to use a topical antibiotic for an infected wound. The nurse knows that this could be inappropriate based on her knowledge of clinical trials and drug data. She can discuss this and offer an alternative dressing.
- The nurse can be asked to carry out a cervical smear test. The carrying out of the test will help the GP reach his cytology targets for the practice. The nurse assesses that the woman did not appreciate what was involved and having discussed it, does not wish to have it done. The assessment process also identifies that she is a virgin and has never managed internal protection with tampons, and has no apparent problems. There are also issues of informed consent and possibly cultural customs. Clinical reasoning with background knowledge of risk factors as well as professional accountability necessitates discussion with the GP, and the woman probably not having the smear test at that time.

Debate is a normal healthy process but needs a productive end and therefore nurses require confidence in articulating their nursing perspective. Disagreements can stimulate creative thought and outcomes. One major area of debate can be the expanding role of nursing.

3.3 Expanding activities

It is by understanding what nursing activities are achieving that the notion of accountability can begin to be addressed (Bottorff and d'Cruz, 1984).

Being an employer does not necessarily mean the GP is aware of the full potential of nursing. The GP's knowledge of nursing may be limited by experience. Paradoxically, there is also expectation that the nurse can expand her skills to almost anything. There is a real possibility that she could become a partner and an independent practitioner.

The legal implications and training requirements for the extending role of the nurse were the subject of a Circular from the Chief Nursing Officer. In it concern was expressed that policies were remote from clinical practice, there was inconsistency in the practice of delegation, inconsistency in the recognition of appropriate training, and no national consensus within the professions.

While the Circular recognised the appropriateness for certain activities to be taught and assessed by the medical profession, it emphasised very clearly that

> the nurse's primary obligation is to the performance of nursing activities that fall within her customary professional role (i.e. those activities for which nurses are prepared in the course of their pre-

registration training and those more specialised activities for which nurses are prepared in their post-registration training). While we welcome the extension of that role in appropriate circumstances, we would not wish it to happen at the expense of the performance of the nurse's customary activities.

(DHSS, 1989)

The implied need within these guidelines was for extended role certificates of competence which further emphasised task competence rather than professional competence. In June 1992, a third edition of the Code of Professional Conduct was published by the UKCC (1992a) and with it a new position statement entitled Scope of Professional Practice (1992b). This latter document replaces the need for extended role certificates and allows individual practitioners to be responsible for negotiating the boundaries of their clinical practice.

In order to bring into proper focus the professional responsibility and consequent accountability of individual practitioners, it is the Council's principles for practice rather than certificates for tasks which should form the basis for adjustments to the scope of practice.

(UKCC, 1992b)

This will not negate the need for continuing post-registration education. Indeed this is recognised and acknowledged in the need to offer evidence of relevant education in order to be entered in the Professional Register and allowed to practice. The development of standards and protocols has been a valuable process in which the nurse and the GP can discuss and negotiate areas of skill and competence and define levels for referral. It is important that the protocols are reviewed regularly to enable the nurse to take on greater responsibility as a result of her experience and continuing education.

3.4 Education

The GP may consider that education and training is the employer's direct responsibility, particularly as part of the responsibilities of delegation. Indeed the Statement on the Terms of Fees and Allowances payable to General Practitioners previously quoted goes some way in confirming this.

Some of the delegated activities may be appropriately taught by the GP providing he himself is competent and up to date with the particular activity. However, with regard to the issue of professional accountability the activity must be set within the context of nursing and not seen as an end activity within itself. Pelvic examination for a well woman check could be an end in itself. However, as part of a nursing activity, the nurse uses this opportunity for assisting the woman to be more aware of her own body and enable her to have control of decisions affecting herself and her lifestyle.

Nursing in general practice was addressed in a specifically related statement issued by the UKCC as a result of the implications of the GP contract. Concern was expressed about the isolation of the nurse but also acknowledged the role.

> their nursing role ... is acceptable, provided that any extension of their role is negotiated with them and builds on their core nursing role. The nurses must be fully prepared in order to practise competently.
>
> (UKCC, 1990)

If the GP takes on the responsibility for the education of 'his nurse', then there is the realistic possibility that she could become his assistant. It has been suggested that even if 'nursing management' is empowering, nurses as a whole are in a subservient position vis a vis administrators, doctors and often other health care staff. One route to empowering is a 'student-centred educational experience' that includes freedom to explore and experiment. Another route for strength is networking with peers for advice and guidance (Chavasse, 1992). Nurses in general practice are a prime example of this as they themselves have formed local groups throughout the UK. These groups exist not only for peer support but have also developed ongoing continuing education programmes. They have also been a significant factor in pressurising educational establishments to offer the National Board approved course and to influence Family Health Services Authorities to offer reimbursement for all or at least some of the fees for educational programmes.

Initiating practice nursing education based on a group and individual negotiated approach to course planning and content was a significant factor in increasing the students' professional confidence. This was demonstrated by more organised approaches to patient care on their return to practice, confidence in their power to alter work patterns, and more realistic terms and conditions of service (Martin, 1988).

Other initiatives have developed from the established courses including Mentorship schemes. It has been perceived that those following the course would benefit from a Mentor who could offer support and guidance and facilitate the practical experience (Richard and Pitman 1989).

It is worth commenting that most of these initiatives are developed and carried out in the nurse's own time and this is a significant factor in demonstrating the commitment, sense of responsibility and enthusiasm of nurses in general practice.

For practice nursing the challenge for professional expertise and the relevant education and training is whether to base it on competence *for* the procedures or competence *in* those procedures as part of nursing. It is perhaps helpful to return to the messages identified in the Damant Report (1990) and reflect on how clinical practice is developing or needs to be developed.

3.5 Professional accountability

If practice nursing is to maintain and enhance its professional creditation and value, it must be regulated within the framework of the Code of Professional Conduct for the Nurse, Midwife and Health Visitor and the Scope of Professional Practice (UKCC, 1992a and b). It is in the knowledge of where the nurse is in relation to exercising accountability that will or will not assist the development of nursing in general practice. Accountability involves responsibility, knowledge and authority and those principles are underlined in the Code of Professional Conduct. The nurse is primarily accountable to the patient, then to her employer and the nursing profession. A significant factor for the nurse in general practice and the employing GP is the opportunity to talk directly about philosophies and expectations of care before agreeing employment. This can result in building up a professional partnership and recognition of each other's specific skills. However, it is also in the framework of management, educational and professional confidence that clinical nursing in general practice has the opportunity to develop.

3.6 Classification of professional status and management styles

The framework below (**Figure 3.1**) offers a classification of professional status and management styles. It suggests when harmony and disagreement can occur.

Authoritative management	
Outcome = Professional disagreement (i)	Outcome = 'employer' dictates the activity to the 'employee' (ii)
Strong professional nursing identity Outcome = Patient centred nursing care (iii)	**Weak professional nursing identity** Outcome = Role and function confusion (iv)
Democratic management	

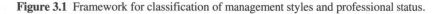

Figure 3.1 Framework for classification of management styles and professional status.

Nursing in general practice could be fitted into any one of the four sections shown in **Figure 3.1**. The challenge for improving clinical practice is in which section that improvement can take place. The following practice example illustrates each of the four sections.

A patient comes to the surgery with inter-menstrual bleeding – she is *very* reluctant to be examined by a male GP.

Section i   The GP requests the nurse to carry out the pelvic examination. The nurse knows that she is unable to make a medical diagnosis, being only competent in recognising a normal pelvis. She cannot justify the patient having two pelvic examinations and therefore refuses.
Result = professional disagreement.

Section ii   The GP requests the nurse to carry out the pelvic examination and she does this.
Result = potential risk of a missed diagnosis and consequent legal and professional implications.

Section iii   The GP acknowledges the nurse's inability to make a medical diagnosis. The nurse uses her professional skill to support and help the patient gain understanding and confidence as the process of diagnosis and potential treatment begins.
Result = complementary care.

Section iv   The GP may persuade the nurse to carry out the pelvic examination because of the patient's reluctance for a male doctor to examine her. For this time only the nurse agrees.
Result = professional uncertainty and possible guilt that inadequate care has been given.

Professional accountability, fully appreciated and acknowledged, results in a legitimate power, and mutual interprofessional acknowledgement of autonomy within that context. This power may relate to expertise, i.e. in a specialist area such as asthma, as well as the 'value' position as a member of staff, with the professional expertise, knowledge and autonomy that implies.

The extent of nursing influence is increasingly demonstrated in relation to setting standards for the control of infection; an area of growing significance with minor surgery and invasive examinations increasing in general practice. Indeed as a member of staff with possibly the most knowledge of control of infection and with the professional accountability to 'safeguard and promote the interests of individual patients and clients' (UKCC, Code of Professional Conduct, 1992a), the nurse has explicit responsibility. Many nurses do take on this responsibility and seek advice from local specialist nurses for control of infection.

Legitimised power is evolved through professional accountability and developing expertise most usually, for nursing in general practice, in a clinical context. This power used confidently and collaboratively is a dynamic force in influencing positive change within health care settings. Evidence suggests that a growing number of nurses are becoming skilled in managing the care of groups of patients such as those with asthma and diabetes, and in health promotion activities. This is in part due to the organisation of general practice and the financial encouragement for developing the management of chronic disease and health promotion and in part due to the nurse herself wishing to develop her role. The challenges for nursing in general practice are to build on the nursing role in what is a medically dominated environment, and to be proactive in seeking out health needs. For example, one can applaud the fact that the target figures for the uptake of cytology and childhood immunisations are met. However, professional responsibility causes one to account for the reasons why the targets do not reach 100%, for example population mobility, clinical contraindications, poor motivation and socioeconomic factors.

3.7 Patient advocacy and empowerment

The nurse also contributes to safeguarding the well being and interests of the practice population within the environment of the practice itself. It is in the knowledge and use of legitimised power that nursing can be valued by the employer, as well as reflect on patients taking responsibility for their own health and provide them with a safe environment in which their health needs are met.

For nurses to empower patients, they need to be confident in their own legitimate power, self awareness and the willingness to release control. There has been discussion of the therapeutic alliance and compliance relationships in the previous chapter.

It is a challenge for nursing in general practice to take on the responsibility to ensure that health needs are met not just by taking a series of measurements but that these measurements are taken within the context of holistic patient care, meeting the health care needs of the person. A number of organisations offer cards or check lists. While these may assist as reminders, there is a danger that, by using them, care can become routine and evaluation is based on completing the cards rather than on the process and outcome of care. Further reference to health promotional activity is made in Chapter 5.

Another challenge for nursing within this context is to ensure that the patient appreciates the implications of tests that have been advised, and has the opportunity to decline. While the GP Contract clearly indicates that health checks should be 'offered', there can remain financial pressure for the GP to ensure that 'the offer' is accepted as, for instance, in the case of cervical smears (DOH, 1990).

Ethical issues arise from the fact that these tasks may be subject to financial incentives but may not necessarily meet the specific needs of the individual. To some degree it can be argued that the GP Contract has resulted from a national perspective of health care needs, for example, targets for cervical cytology and child immunisations have been an incentive to improve the nation's health and prevent disease. However, health promotion clinics could be set up not because of a perceived and identified need, but because of available staff and financial incentive. By 1992 concerns about the lack of strategy and the increasing emphasis on structure had led to a temporary moratorium on health promotion clinics.

Nursing in general practice, because of its potentially medically dominated environment, must develop the identification and meeting of patients' needs with or without the GP's medical diagnosis and contractual responsibilities. Indeed lack of hierarchical control as in the Health Authority set-up means that the work can develop according to the needs of patients and not within a structured system and indeed this is happening.

> By negotiating their own role (practice nurses) can question the reasoning behind each aspect of their work; for example, community needs, finance available and personal competence.
>
> (Peachey, 1987)

Professionalism can improve service through clinical expertise and knowledge and by the position that knowledge and expertise validates and accredits. It is through the nurse acknowledging clinical competence and limitations that GPs can appreciate nursing skills and professional development can take place.

3.8 Skill mix and appropriate use of resources

It is in this context that nursing in general practice needs to address itself, particularly in exploring how outcomes of patient care match the clinical skills of the nurse. A greater understanding is needed to identify the relationship between skill mix, quality of care and patient outcomes.

For example, taking a health check: a trained helper could weigh, measure and carry out a urinalysis, allowing the practice nurse more time to interpret and discuss the implications of the test results with the patient.

A review of the literature about skill mix in nursing recognises the complexities of professionalism and resource management. Skill mix has been defined as:

> the balance between trained and untrained, qualified and unqualified, and supervisory and operative staff within a service area as well as different staff groups. The optimum skill mix is achieved when a desired standard of service is provided at the minimum cost, which is consistent with the efficient deployment of trained, qualified and supervisory personnel and the maximisation of contributions from all staff.
>
> (North East Thames Regional Health Authority, 1992)

Clinical grading is one component of a wider skill mix exercise. In general practice this has been addressed more towards the qualifications and length of professional experience rather than the job itself. The absence of a specific body of knowledge which underpins practice nursing, the variations in practice and the individual employment of nurses create problems for the development of a 'blanket' policy. More specific guidelines are being prepared by Family Health Service Authorities, based on the recommendations issued by the RCN and DOH. It is, however, important to note that GPs can pay their employees whatever is negotiated; it is the level of reimbursement by FHSAs that may relate more to national guidelines. The flexibility and functions within nursing in general practice are one of its main attractions.

On the other hand, there is little point in having two nurses both having an advanced level of knowledge in the same area within the one practice setting. There is still a clear need from a managerial view to:

> identify procedures which require a nursing qualification and to allow others to undertake the procedures requiring less skills. From this point of view, both substitution and an expanded role are legitimate, provided that the procedures are within the capabilities of the performer.
>
> (Gibbs *et al.*, 1991).

3.9 Documentation

The emphasis in this chapter has been to challenge nursing in general practice in developing its clinical approaches to care. This needs to be demonstrated not only by actual practice and outcomes but also in writing, as part of professional accountability. One of the potential limitations is that nursing notes are combined with medical notes and these are often kept in Lloyd George envelopes in which space is limited. A4-size notes are used in some practices but this is not common. Another alternative is to enter the consultation details on a computer data base. Provided there is confidentiality, storage and back-up available to conserve the input, there is no problem with the principle but limitations can occur because of lack of ability to demonstrate a nursing plan and outcome. It is obviously ideal to share the same notes with the GP in order to avoid duplication and for each discipline to gain from each other's perspectives. However, not all GPs may appreciate this and anecdotal evidence suggests that if the notes are 'too long' the GP may complain. General practice has obvious advantages in relation to hospital organisation or other community nursing, where each discipline keeps its own notes. Perhaps the best way forward is for the patient to hold the records – something which is already being done for child health care and maternity care. The challenge is for the nurse to write relevant information succinctly and to ensure that the nursing perspective and framework is identified in whatever type of notes are being used. Earlier reference to nursing frameworks has stressed further significance to the appropriate documentation of care.

To improve and value clinical practice, nursing in general practice needs to evaluate both the process and outcomes of care and to ensure that it is the nurses who determine their own potential and limitations. Professionalism demands self regulation but also recognition and use of skills. This will require setting and monitoring of standards both at national and local levels. National standards have been developed by the RCN Practice Nurse Association as part of the Standards of Care project.

Documentation can be used to effect appropriate nursing and resource management. It is also implicit to evaluate practice critically as part of the management process. These aspect s are further addressed in Chapter 6.

Summary

Nursing in general practice makes its contribution to community health care as clinical practice continues to move forward firmly rooted in the context of nursing. This is developed by using clinical reasoning based on a framework of nursing independent but 'complementary to medicine'.

Nursing in general practice is a discrete area of practice meeting the health needs of the practice population. In part this has been due to the GP Contract and its commitment to preventive health care, and in part due to the initiatives of GPs and nurses who recognise the value of shared and collaborative care.

Not least, it is the patients who will appreciate the choice of whom they can consult. The nurses in this area can confidently move forward, their activities based within the scope of professional practice and accountability.

References

Bottorff J and d'Cruz J (1984), Notions of nursing. *Journal of Advanced Nursing*, **9**(6), pp. 549–553.

Carnevali D L, Mitchell P H, Woods N F and Tanner C A (1984), *Diagnostic Reasoning in Nursing*. Philadelphia: Lippincott.

Chavasse J (1992), New dimensions of empowerment in nursing. Guest editorial. *Journal of Advanced Nursing*, **17**(1), pp. 1–2.

Clarke J (1992), *The Value of Nursing*. London: Royal College of Nursing.

Cumberlege J (1986), *Report of the Community Nursing Review 'Neighbourhood Nursing – A Focus for Care'*. London: HMSO.

Damant M (1990), *Report of the Review Group for the Education and Training for Practice Nursing 'The Challenges of Primary Health Care in the 1990s'*. London: (ENB).

De La Cuesta C (1979), In: Hollingworth S (1986), The nursing process: implications for curriculum planning. *Journal of Advanced Nursing*, **11**(2), 212.

DHSS (1989), *The Extending Role of the Nurse*. PL/CMO (89) 7, PL/CNO (89) 10. DHSS, London.

DOH and Welsh Office (1990), *General Medical Services. Statements of fees and allowances payable to General Medical Practitioners in England and Wales from 1 April 1990*. London: HMSO.

Gambrill E (1980), In: Fry J (ed) *Primary Care*. London: Heinemann Medical Books.

Gibbs I, McCaughan D and Griffiths M (1991), Skill mix in nursing: a selective review of the literature. *Journal of Advanced Nursing*, **16**(2), pp. 242–249.

Martin C (1988), *An Innovative Approach to the Professional Preparation of Practice Nurses Demonstrated in a Learning Package and a Short Course*. Unpublished MPhil thesis, University of London.

McFarlane J and Castledine G (1982), *A Guide to the Practice of Nursing Using the Nursing Process*. St Louis: C V Mosby.

North East Thames Regional Health Authority (1992), *Skill Mix and Reprofiling: a Guide for RCN Members*. London: Royal College of Nursing.

Peachey M (1987), A GP Employee? The case for Nursing Times. *Nursing Times*, **83**(17), p. 34.

Pembrey S (1984), Nursing care: professional progress. *Journal of Advanced Nursing*, **9**(6), pp. 539–546.

Reedy B (1972), The general practice nurse I. *Update*, **3**, pp. 75–78.

Reedy B, Metcalf A, de Roumanie M and Newell D (1980), A comparison of the activities and opinions of attached and employed nurses in general practice. *Journal of the Royal College of General Practitioners,* **30**, pp. 483–489.

Richard S and Pitman B (1989), Mentorship scheme for practice nurse course. *Practice Nurse,* **Sept 89**, pp. 179–182.

RCGP (1972), In: Driver P (1986), *A Trainee in General Practice.* Leighton Buzzard, Bedfordshire: Association of Health Centre and Practice Administrators (AHCPA).

UKCC (1990), *Statement on Practice Nurses and Aspects of the New GP Contract.* London: UKCC.

UKCC (1992), *Code of Professional Conduct for the Nurse, Midwife and Health Visitor, 3rd edn.* London: UKCC.

UKCC (1992), *The Scope of Professional Practice.* London: UKCC.

Warrier S (1992), *Nursing in Primary Care. A Profile of Practice Nurses in South East Thames.* Research undertaken on behalf of Regional Directorate of Nursing and Quality. South East Thames Regional Health Authority.

4 Team working

Team working, or some form of cooperation between people, has always been a feature of primary care. The district nurse, the midwife and the health visitor have liaised with GPs to a greater or lesser extent. Nurses as employees of general practice have had close contact with the GP and many have established a special working relationship. Since the mid-1970s, however, there has been an increasing emphasis on more formal links between health professionals working in the community. The term primary health care team has been used for some time to refer to doctors, nurses and other practice staff working in general practice. But what many might question is that although there may have been some form of cooperation between individuals this has not been real team working, rather an informal network. The degree of joint planning and discussion of care management may have been determined by the personalities of the people involved. The recent White Papers (Working for Patients, 1989a; Caring for People, 1989b) have both put considerable emphasis on team working either directly or by implication. There is emphasis on integration of services avoiding overlap, and on cost-effective practice and services that reflect the health needs of the communities being served.

In this chapter it is intended to discuss briefly the recent government initiatives and consider different types of teams. Definitions of 'team' and 'team working' will be stated, and principles of team work and nursing in general practice as part of a multiprofessional service will be discussed. Finally, barriers and opportunities will be considered with some examples from practice.

4.1 Recent government initiatives

The recent government initiatives have the intention of a needs-led service with patients receiving appropriate care when they require it. At the heart of Caring for People (1989) are core assessment, care management and the notion of joint care plans. There is an explicit expectation of cooperation across agencies with cooperation between both health and social care in terms of care objectives. Social services is the lead agency, holding the budget for social provision and expected to coordinate social provision in relation to health provision. Central to Working for Patients is the role of primary care. The general practice is the focus of community health provision with clear implications for team working as a mechanism for coordinating provision. The GP Contract has obliged GPs to harness resources in order to meet targets, however the validity of the targets set is open to question. In this context for both contemporary health and social care we are operating in an environment where the expectation is for maximum cost-effective use of resources, that is targeting need in as precise a fashion as possible and serving that need in the most efficient way. Team working is being seen as essential in terms of coordinating human resources, reducing duplication of input and targeting appropriate output. In Chapter 5 health promotion is suggested to be an activity shared by all health professionals. The implication of efficient team working is that one health professional takes a leading role. However, there is an assumption underlying the emphasis that team working is both more effective and more efficient, although there is no objective evidence to support this assumption. The observation has been made that at present there is confusion about what constitutes a primary health care team, and we lack agreed criteria for evaluating the performance of the team (Jones, 1992). We hope that team working is efficient.

There are organisational issues that can hinder partnership between professions working from a general practice in terms of multiple employers and multiple provider units. A recent editorial in the *British Journal of General Practice* suggests that there needs to be very clear thinking about organisational models adopted in the future (Salisbury, 1991). Referring particularly to the working arrangements between GPs and nurses, the government intention is that any organisational structure of nursing services needs to focus on primary care. There are further issues of employer–employee arrangements between nurses and GPs that will be discussed in a later chapter.

The distinction has been made between single disciplinary teams such as a team of health visitors, multidisciplinary or multiprofessional teams and multi-agency teams (Poulton, 1991). The focus of this chapter will be the multiprofessional team, and this will be multiprofessional in terms of professions other than nursing, although barriers between different branches of community nursing will be briefly considered.

4.2 Definitions of teams and team working

There are many definitions of teams and team working. All emphasise working together but can make different points. Barber and Kratz (1980) offered the following definition:

> Team care means that people from different disciplines work together in providing care for patients. In this case the context is primary care or general practice, with the implication that team care has advantages over individual professionals working on their own.

The primary health care team was defined in the Harding Report (1981) as being:

> ... an interdependent group of GPs, secretaries/receptionists, health visitors, district nurses and midwives who share a common purpose and responsibility each member clearly understanding his/her function and those of other members, so that they all pool skills and knowledge to provide an effective primary health care service.

The definition of members needs to be extended to include not just nurses working in general practice but therapists who may now be included in the team. The emphasis on interdependence is useful, as it acknowledges that no one profession can serve all the functions required of primary care; rather there are specialist inputs dependent on requirements. A further definition that is cited in

Poulton (1991) comes from the then National Health Service Training Authority now the National Health Service Training Directorate.

> A team is a collection of individuals who have an explicit reason for working together, and are in need of each other's abilities and skills.

This definition implies a clear purpose for the team and again mutual benefits from coordinating skills.

Effective team working has been suggested to:

- Increase productivity.
- Improve the quality of output.
- Enhance working relationships.
- Be a very cost-effective use of employee time (Munro, 1991).

This implies commitment on the part of team members. It also implies that people need to meet as a team on a regular basis, have clear and agreed team roles and a clearly defined shared purpose or goal. All these principles are implicit within the definitions above. A team may initially form in response to a specific problem, and as a consequence of that experience the benefits and value of that way of working is appreciated. Many primary health care teams have started in this way.

There can also be teams within teams. For example, within the primary care team there may be project teams set up for a particular purpose. There may be a team comprising a doctor, a nurse and the practice manager to organise and implement information technology within the practice. Many books have been written about teamwork in terms of management and there are distance learning materials to help practices to organise their teams in the most effective fashion (Adair, 1986; Munro, 1991).

The role of individual members of the team may vary with the task being undertaken, not in a hierarchical fashion. In many instances a key worker will be nominated by the group. A key worker in the case of patient care will be the team member nominated to have the closest contact with the patient because of their particular skills in relation to patient need. They will draw on the skills of others as appropriate, thus reducing overlap in activity and targeting input that the patient needs, when they need it. There are similarities to the concept of care management in social care as both key workers and care managers are responsible for the coordination of input, ensuring that, as far as possible, it matches the patient or client need.

Protocols offer the opportunity for team work to be demonstrated in reality. This requires negotiation between team members, e.g. nurse and doctor, and is necessarily time consuming. The nurse needs to identify her function within the bounds of that protocol and ensure that the patients' nursing needs are being addressed. This is a practical example of clinical reasoning.

4.3 The multiprofessional team and nursing in general practice

In Chapter 3 the concept of legitimate power was introduced. In a climate of increasing accountability clear definitions of role, function and responsibility are required, with a definite understanding of the accompanying knowledge, skills and values. Such a clear understanding allows respect between the team members. Nursing in general practice can be suggested to be central to the primary health care team because of the critical role in health promotion and the management of chronic disorders. The nurse frequently holds the patient together, calling on specialist input as required, for example the asthma clinic. The nurse monitors, advises and educates. However, the specialist input of the physiotherapist may be called upon to give specific advice on breathing and exercise. Nursing can facilitate both the integration of services as a team member and the continuity of care. The system of recording is, however, critical. Recording to ensure both legal requirements and continuity of care needs to be a precise record of both assessment and intervention. What is implicit in team working is that the record is shared and accessible to all the team members.

What are the potential problems of team working? There can be moral and ethical dilemmas, for example with confidentiality. Computers can be programmed to allow differential access to team members, but how much patient confidence should be shared with other team members in order to manage a situation effectively? Decisions about disclosure of potentially confidential information by necessity must be a matter of professional judgement. There can also be problems of collusion, against the patient or with the patient. Collusion against the patient can occur when the team consider they know what is best, regardless of the individual's wishes. This may be in terms of long term planning involving relatives and residential care. Collusion by one member of the team with the patient against another team member can also occur. Imagine a situation where the doctor has prescribed medication for a patient with a mental health problem. The patient has been given clear advice about how to take the medication, when to expect an effect and to persist even though there is no immediate benefit. Another team member disagrees with this form of treatment and advises the patient accordingly, suggesting that they should ask for a change of therapy. What is the moral position? The doctor has made what is considered to be the best decision based on expectations of likely outcome, yet another team member is undermining this decision. On what basis? There are no absolute criteria against which a treatment decision of this nature can be made; the doctor considers that he/she has acted on the best available information. This is a problem because if the other professional is not party to further information, this is simply a competing opinion.

A further challenge for team working is the traditional doctor–nurse, male–female dominance. In reality there are differences in the level of medical and nursing education and differences in the levels of decisions made. But for team working to happen an ability to take the lead where appropriate and to allow others to take it when it is not, is critical. In summary, there is an apparent consensus that team working is an effective and satisfying organisational strategy. The principles are to agree common goals, clearly define the roles, and cater for group, individual and task needs (Munro, 1991).

4.4 Opportunities and barriers

Barriers to communication can occur simply because of geography. GPs communicated more frequently with health visitors and district nurses who were attached and housed at the same location than those who were housed at another location (Bond et al., 1985). Barriers to cooperation between health visitors and district nurses were found to be failures of communication and misunderstanding of role (Poulton, 1991). Effective systems of communication are suggested to be critical for effective team working, as has been found in a study of older people (Giarchi, 1988). At the professional level all practitioners can be guilty of delaying referrals at the appropriate time. This may be due to an inadequate assessment or to a lack of knowledge, or to the influence of negative attitudes. For whatever reason this may cause the patient to suffer unnecessarily. Furthermore, inappropriate intervention may 'muddy the water' for other professionals who follow. This is a phenomenon to which attention has been drawn, particularly in the situation of child abuse and family violence. On a very practical level there are issues of space and time. A room is needed for team meetings and punctuality is critical where time is money and patient needs are the overriding consideration. For many nurses barriers can arise due to part-time employment; if there is a lack of commitment these barriers may be insuperable. Further to the last point, many practices employ several nurses on a part-time basis and it is quite possible for there to be no overlap within the working day. The potential for professional isolation is a real issue and this perpetuates the isolation referred to in Chapter 1. Developing a strategy for allowing this team to meet and negotiating overlap is a way of overcoming the difficulty. It provides an opportunity for considering nursing as a whole within general practice.

Potential barriers can be related to aspects of personality. Where a team member is very dominant and unable to allow others to contribute in any way, other than subserviently, there are problems. For some people experiencing a change of role and adapting to change may take time. There are clear issues surrounding the nature of employment; these may or may not be a problem, depending on the attitudes of the team involved. Just as excessive dominance is a problem so is a lack of assertiveness. If assertiveness can be equated in this context with confidence, it may be linked to educational opportunity. The differences in educational opportunities between medicine and nursing were referred to earlier. Differences in intellectual ability that result from different educational opportunities can pose a barrier to the negotiation processes. Extending educational opportunities can also threaten some traditional relationships.

General practitioners undergo a complete medical training and then a further period of vocational training before becoming fully fledged practitioners. As a consequence they have had the opportunity to develop their clinical reasoning skills in general practice. Until recently nurses in general practice had little educational opportunity to prepare them for their role in general practice. The standard of pre-registration training has been raised recently to diploma level and student nurses are indeed students and no longer apprentices. This gives them the opportunity to develop the clinical and intellectual skills needed to identify and justify good nursing practice. Nurses who have gone before have had to develop these skills more fully after qualification. A Royal College of Nursing publication addressing future nursing education and training suggested that nurses at that time were crying out for time to think and reason (Judge, 1988).

The educational provision for nursing within the context of rapidly changing primary health care deserves careful consideration, and there are many developments in different parts of the United Kingdom. Nurses in general practice have been very vigorous and active in seeking educational opportunities. They have also been vigorous in developing interest groups that can give peer support to less experienced members and peers can assist in the development of clinical skills. Departments of General Practice are uniquely placed to promote multiprofessional education and short training courses for the whole team, for example study days on clinical audit where there is a mutual investment in the improvement of care and the introduction of new ways of working. In a recent Royal College of General Practitioners Occasional Paper the growth and importance of team working has been emphasised, as have multiprofessional educational initiatives (Pereira Gray, 1992).

Opportunities have been taken in different areas to develop teams both within primary health care and also across health and social care agencies. Project work has taken place in East Sussex in anticipation of the full implementation of the Community Care Act (Murphy and Rodrigues, 1992). Care managers have been located in general practice and methods for joint assessment and joint care planning have been developed and were being tested at that time. Whether or not this is carried forward is dependent on finance.

Further examples of cooperation between social services and primary health care are now numerous, but for the clients and patients to appreciate a real benefit, input needs to be coordinated through collaborative teamwork. Practice reports need to reflect the wide range of diverse skills being offered by team members, diverse skills that all contribute to effective patient care, but need to be made known in order that patients may gain maximum benefit. A study exploring usefulness of a practice brochure that described the primary health care team and what could be offered found that there was a significantly greater use of non-doctor members of the team by patients who had read the brochure compared with those who had not (Marsh, 1980).

There are interesting developments in Europe for team working in Primary Health Care. At a recent conference in Finland papers were presented which focused on the relationship between health needs and the multiprofessional expertise required to address them. From the assessment of need multi-professional and single professional involvement was identified (European Network for Multiprofessional Education Annual Conference, 1992). The presentations suggested that professional identity is defined, in part, by the contribution made to the team.

Professional identity of individual team members is essential for effective team working and is implicit within the multidisciplinary structure of primary care. A further essential criterion is commitment to the philosophy and objectives of the team to which one belongs. Opportunities to meet need to be created in order to build team spirit. Appropriate and possibly rotating leadership is important and implies that team members value each other. An example of such a team could be the practice team setting up a system for audit. This not only involves administrative decisions but also professional decisions that are client centred together with a commitment by the team to learn this process together.

Summary

Nurses in general practice have always been part of the primary health care team and recent social policy has put a very high emphasis on team working in health and social care. Team working is viewed as being critical to an effective, coordinated and integrated service that makes the best use of scarce resources.

An effective team needs effective communication strategies. It needs to meet regularly, and each of the members needs to have a clear understanding of the roles, functions and skills of their colleagues and agreed clear team roles. The purposes and goals of the team need to be clear and shared. Education needs to cater for team working if it is to succeed in realising policy intentions. Although many untested assumptions do underlie the social policy, nurses in general practice can take the lead in helping to develop team working further within their practice. It is also critical that nurses in general practice build their own uniprofessional team in order to enhance nursing within the practice.

References

Adair J (1986), *Effective Teambuilding*. London: Gower.

Barber J H and Kratz C (1980), *Towards Team Care*. Edinburgh: Churchill Livingstone.

Bond J, Cartilidge A M, Gregson B A, Philips P R, Bolam F and Gill K M (1985), A Study of Interprofessional Collaboration in Primary Health Care Organisations. *Health Care Research Unit,* 2, 27, University of Newcastle Upon Tyne.

DOH (1989a), *Working for Patients: A Review of the National Health Service.* London: HMSO.

DOH (1989b), *Caring for People. Community Care in the Next Decade and Beyond.* London: HMSO.

European Network For Development of Multiprofessional Education in Health Sciences (1992), *Challenges of Multiprofessional Training for Management and Training in Health Care.* Annual Conference 10–12 June, Tampere, Finland.

Giarchi G (1988), *Communicating Information about Older People.* Devon Social Services: Plymouth.

Harding W G (1981), *A Report of a Joint Working Group of the Standing Medical Advisory Committee and the Standing Nursing and Midwifery Advisory Committee 'The Primary Health Care Team'.* London: DHSS.

Jones RVH (1992), Teamwork in Primary Care: How Much do we Know About it? *Journal of Interprofessional Care,* **6**(1), pp. 25–29.

Judge H (1988), *The Education of Nurses: A New Dispensation.* Commission on Nursing Education, Royal College of Nursing of the United Kingdom.

Marsh G N (1980), The practice brochure: a patient's guide to team care. *British Medical Journal,* **281**(9), pp. 730–732.

Munro K (1991), *Teamwork in Practice.* London: BMS College for Continuing Medical Education.

Murphy G and Rodrigues L (1992), Joint assessment for community care in East Sussex. *Primary Health Care Management,* **2**, pp. 10–11.

Pereira Gray D (1992), *Planning Primary Care. A discussion document.* Occasional Paper 57. London: Royal College of General Practitioners.

Poulton B (1991), Does your team really work? *Primary Health Care,* **1**, pp. 11–14.

Salisbury C (1991), Working in partnership with nurses. *British Journal of General Practice,* **October**, pp. 398–399.

5 Health promotion

Health promotion has played a significant part in confirming the role of the nurse in general practice. As a result of a greater commitment to it in the GP Contract, and the recognition of nursing skills, the number of nurses in general practice rose significantly between 1989 and 1990. Indeed nurses in general practice have demonstrated innovative and dynamic approaches to health promotion. However, the emphasis on health promotion in the GP Contract has raised criticisms both because of the fiscal arrangements within the Contract and the limitations within the context of the practice population. This chapter offers a perspective of the evolving commitment to health promotion through Government strategies and the nursing profession. It helps the nurse in general practice to consider her actual and potential role within the total perspective of health promotion and to gain some understanding of the issues surrounding health choices for the patient. There are many resources that assist the nurse to identify, plan and evaluate health promotional activities although it is not practical or relevant for these to be discussed in this book. Chapter 1 has already outlined the increasing significance of the promotion of health and prevention of ill health in primary health care to which nursing in general practice has made significant contributions.

5.1 The concept of health

Assumptions based on traditional paradigms of health have identified it as the absence of disease. Care is aimed at curing or relieving the symptoms of the disease process. However, shifts in concepts of health have emerged to equate health with a positive lifestyle, self responsibility and life satisfaction. The following definition has been suggested:

> health is the effective functioning of self-care resources which ensure the operation and adequacy of self-care actions. Self-care resources would include knowledge, skills and attitudes. An example of a 'health attitude' is that life is seen as worthwhile, under control and having predictability. The self-care actions of individuals would be goal directed behaviours required to retain, maintain or promote one's physical, psychosocial and spiritual functioning.
>
> (Payne, 1983)

This shift to maintaining lifestyle normality is reflected in a number of discussion documents particularly related to primary health care in the community. The Thirtieth World Health Assembly in 1977 decided to adopt 'health for all' as the main social target of governments and WHO for the coming decades; it was seen as a standard of health that would permit people to lead a socially and economically productive life (Mahler, 1979). In the following year an opportune and important initiative took place at the International Conference on Primary Care held at Alma-Ata sponsored by WHO and UNICEF. The conference issued a Declaration which reiterated that primary health care was the key to attaining a desired level of health throughout the world (Reid, 1979). The initial emphasis is therefore on community involvement and community services rather than on the more specialised and expensive aspects of health care. The aim announced by the conference was 'health for all by the year 2000' (WHO, 1978). Strategies to achieve this aim are based on international and local initiatives offering a diversity of approaches relevant to specific needs. The implications of monitoring and evaluation are obvious together with the need to exchange information at the various levels.

In the UK this shift was seen in two discussion documents issued in 1986: *Neighbourhood Nursing – a Focus for Care*: Report of the Community Nursing Review (DHSS, 1986a) and *Project 2000 UKCC: a New Preparation for Practice (UKCC, 1986).*

The first document's term of reference was to study nursing services provided outside hospital. The Review team was concerned primarily with the needs of the consumer and not with the needs of the service. People wanted information about health care which they could easily understand and relate to themselves; what could be done to prevent ill health and promote good health; the support and advisory services provided by nurses and doctors; and how to make use of those services.

The second document identified one of the trends of health care in the next decade to be an emphasis on health promotion and disease prevention and on primary health care in the community.

It is with this emphasis that it proposed the initial common foundation programmes for nurse training should be based on health and *not* illness.

The Government also appreciates that primary health care plays a key role not only in the treatment of disease, but also in maintenance and promotion of health. The Government's aim to improve services for the public includes in its key objectives:

> to make services more responsive to the consumer; to raise standards
> of care; to promote health and prevent illness.

(DHSS, 1986b)

The role of the nurse as identified in these documents is not only with the sick person but also with health promotion for the well person and maintaining health in the presence of a chronic disease. In this respect there is also the need to encourage compliance in the individual who may not perceive themselves in need of care. An example is seen in the person with stable diabetes mellitus who perceives himself as well, and may not appreciate that the regular periodic care anticipates potential problems that can be identified on tests and questioning.

5.2 The emerging significance of health promotion

The role and significance of health promotion for nursing is reiterated in later documents including 'A Strategy for Nursing' (DOH Nursing Division, 1989) and a series from the Royal College of Nursing on issues in nursing and health. The former stresses the importance of partnership with other health professionals but also points to the main role of community nurses to be to:

> change attitudes, making people better aware of active health promotion and self care, and offering to those who are already coping with problems to the best of their ability, the practical assistance and advice which will enable them to do so more effectively.
>
> (DOH Nursing Division, 1989).

The latter document identifies the nature of nursing to be: 'helping people – as individuals, families and communities in the achievement and maintenance of good health' (RCN, 1992).

Health promotion, highlighted in the 1987 White Paper 'Promoting Better Health', forms a significant part of the GP Contract. In this there is a major shift towards a range of preventive activities in general practice. Health promotion is explicitly identified in the context of health checks for defined groups in the population, health promotion clinics to cover specific or general topics in relation to anticipatory and preventive care and payments for achieving target rates for the uptake of child immunisation and cytology.

A further commitment to health is seen in the White Paper 'The Health of the Nation', published in 1992. This sets out a strategy for England selecting the initial five areas for action which are:

● Coronary heart disease and stroke.
● Cancers, particularly lung, breast, cervical and skin cancers.
● Mental illness and particularly to reduce the suicide rates.
● Human immunodeficiency virus (HIV)/acquired immune deficiency syndrome (AIDS) and sexual health.
● Accidents – the most common cause of death in young people.

All these areas are associated with great need, identified risk factors and have the greatest scope for making cost effective improvements in the overall health of the country. The White Paper reiterates the need and importance for 'active partnerships between many organisations and individuals who can come together to help improve health ...' (DOH, 1992). The emphasis is on enabling all concerned to focus their efforts on common objectives and provide a yardstick for measurement.

Action should take place in a wide variety of settings. The strategy includes setting the framework for monitoring, development and review. It also sets the responsibility for these activities within the setting of primary health care.

The other UK countries have also developed similar strategies.

5.3 The potential of health promotion for nursing in general practice

Into this scenario, nursing in general practice adds its role. Although the GP Contract emphasises increased commitment to health promotion, nurses in general practice were already involved in this activity.

The review of practice nursing reiterates that competencies in nursing in general practice should reflect skills in conducting health promotion activities and health education and enabling patients/clients to maximise their health potential (Damant, 1990).

In the 'Standards for Care' document for nursing in general practice – the topic of health promotion is specifically focused in the introduction and recognises that much of the work of the practice nurse involves important steps in preventive health care and health education. At the same time it is recognised that the autonomy of the patient and community participation in health matters should be encouraged (RCN, 1991).

Within the context of health promotion the nurse has the opportunity to offer advice, explanation or referral to the GP or possibly another agency (depending on the degree of professional autonomy). The 1990 GP Contract enabled the confirmation of the nursing role in health promotion. The role and function could be established by means of developing standards and protocols agreed with the GP. These set parameters for care and identify acceptable ranges for test results. (The results of the consultation may be recorded either in the notes or, more frequently, a specific record card may be used which is then inserted into the notes envelope.) Documentation is also the means of evaluating and auditing the quality of care offered to the patient.

5.4 Evaluation and audit

While auditing examines whether or not quality has been achieved, evaluation also includes subjective perceptions and opinions not only by the clinicians but also by the patient. Both together offer the opportunity to assure quality care.

It is perhaps helpful to compare the definitions of nursing and medical audit and to consider their implications when evaluating health promotion activities as a practice team.

Nursing forms:

> part of the quality assurance cycle. It incorporates systematic and critical analyses by nurse, midwives and health visitors, in conjunction with other staff, of the planning, delivery and evaluation of nursing and midwifery care, in terms of their use and resources and the outcomes for patients/clients and introduces appropriate changes in response to that analysis.

> (NHS Management Executive, 1991)

A Department of Health working paper defines medical audit as:

> The systematic, critical analysis of the quality of medical care, including the procedures used for diagnosis and treatment, the use of resources, and the resulting outcome and quality of life for the patient.
>
> (Working Paper 6, DOH, 1989)

While both definitions are concerned with similar outcomes, it is the approach that reflects the different practitioner perspectives. However, as desired health outcomes cannot be achieved by one person and because collaborative and shared care is part of general practice, it can be argued that the term clinical audit should be used. If protocols and standards are agreed, then into that can be built agreed clinical audit methodology. The limitations of documentation do encourage the tendency to audit only quantitative concrete data relating to such things as:

● Numbers attending clinics.
● Numbers requiring follow-up.
● Alterations in lifestyle and/or recordings.

The qualitative aspect is more difficult to record and document but, nevertheless, needs to be addressed. It includes the quality of technical care, interpersonal skills and the amenities and environment where the care is provided (Donabedian, 1989).

Evaluation is an integral part of professional accountability and the nurse in general practice needs to reflect on how both the process and outcome of evaluation can be demonstrated in clinical activity practice and in documentation.

5.5 Limitations of the GP Contract for health promotion

Criticism has been levelled at the GP Contract which emphasises a task centred approach and does not offer a more holistic approach to health promotion, which is a complex concept as Smail (1990) illustrates.

> One of the targets for health promotion is indeed – as the new contract suggests – the improvement of lifestyle. However, lifestyle is not synonymous with health behaviour, it consists of the interplay between living conditions, in the wide sense, and individual patterns of behaviour, as determined by social cultural factors and personal characteristics.

On the other hand, health promotion could be seen as imposed and reactive to a perceived fiscal contractual responsibility. It has the implications for assuming the patient/client is following an 'unhealthy lifestyle' and imposes certain lifestyle changes which may or may not be acceptable or even possible.

Criticism has also been levelled at nursing in general practice itself in regard to health promotional activities, both in its limitations and lack of skills. This is partly due to the fact that it is seen as part of a medical framework and to the 'task' oriented approach within the GP Contract. The recognition of health promotion is welcomed but can be criticised. Four interrelated adverse consequences have been suggested:

- Opportunistic health checks are not encouraged because of the fiscal arrangements for health promotion clinics.
- People in more affluent (and healthier) social classes tend to take up the offers for health checks.
- Team work with other health workers who may have more expertise is not encouraged. For example, the health visitor employed by the Authority/Trust may be more skilled in running a smoking cessation group but the Contract encourages the practice to set up a separate group in order to claim their fee.
- Health promotion requires close collaboration between all agencies such as voluntary agencies, local authorities, etc., and this is not supported in the Contract (Griffiths, 1990).

By June 1992 widespread concern about the context of health promotion clinics within general practice resulted in a fact sheet from the National Health Service Management Executive advising that health promotional activities are to be set in a 'framework of national and local priorities, informed by the Health of the Nation initiative and equivalent Scottish and Welsh strategic guidance'.

It is envisaged that 'a range of approaches should be offered while ensuring that resources are focused on activities of greatest benefit to patients. There will also be an organisational framework to enable a more predictable allocation of resources ... and promote equality of access to health promotion' (NHS Management Executive, 1992).

The changes that took place from July 1993, with three developmental bands to allow practices to progress from a minimal to maximum approach to health promotion. In line with the Health of the Nation Strategy, coronary heart disease is suggested as the first priority area. Chronic disease management is a separate provision, asthma and diabetes being specifically named.

5.6 The context of health promotion

It is essential that the context of nursing in general practice is considered within the definitions and models for health promotion and that the nurse in general practice can identify her role and scope of professional practice within that framework.

A widely accepted definition of the scope of health promotion has been described as 'comprising efforts to enhance positive health and prevent ill-health through the overlapping areas of health education, prevention and health protection' (Tannahill, 1985).

Health education is familiar to most nurses but is also perhaps the area that is most widely interpreted. One impression may be that it is 'telling people what to do'. However, this goes a very little way in empowering the recipient to have the knowledge, skills, motivation and confidence to make informed choices about healthy lifestyles, the underlying aim of education. It takes time for preparation, communication and assessment of learning and of course is not limited to a one to one basis but is extended to group activities and to communities. Health education is a participative exercise between the provider and the recipients.

Prevention. Central to this is the reduction of risks influencing the occurrence of disease process, injury or illness. Prevention incorporates such activities as immunisation and screening. This is clearly identified within the GP Contract with the financial incentive to meet cervical cytology and child immunisation targets. The breast mammography screening programme is another example of this activity.

Health protection is the evolving role of public health. It has been defined as 'legal and fiscal controls, other regulations and policies and voluntary codes of practice aimed at the enhancement of positive health and the prevention of ill-health (Tannahill, 1985). Such activities as national no-smoking days, non-smoking areas in public places and tax levies on alcohol and cigarettes contribute to health protection.

Within the framework Tannahill suggests the main sections overlap. These sub-sections are concerned more with the process of health promotion. **Figure 5.1** illustrates how these processes influence and result in the interrelation of all areas. The central process to all health promotional activities is the efforts aimed at creating an environment in which health choices can be made. This turns the activity to lobbying influential people to creating a social climate in which the public can find health choices easier to make (Tannahill, 1985).

The following example applies the framework to child immunisation and may help the nurse in general practice to reflect on her role in such an example as well as appreciate the influence of other resources and factors influencing the uptake.

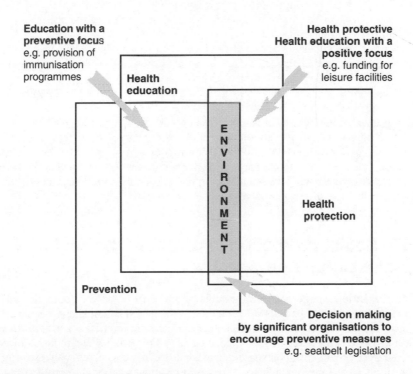

Figure 5.1 A framework for health promotion.

Health education prevention	It is through health education that the mother appreciates the value of prevention and brings her child for immunisation.
Health protective health education	Advertising and marketing the immunisation clinic gives the mother further encouragement to attend. Marketing knowledge may result in the clinic being held at the same time as the 'Well baby' clinic to achieve a higher attendance as well as making use of available resources.
Preventive health protection	Financial incentive is an additional encouragement to the GP to ensure the children in the practice receive their immunisations.
The environment	This is influenced by the Government's commitment to releasing funding for the incentives. It comes as a result of both public health data and pressure to prevent childhood diseases and reduce mortality and morbidity.

It can be seen from this example and application that health promotion is a complex activity involving not only the provider and consumer but also a wider input on a national basis. It is also clear that the skills of education, marketing, politicising and financial management are all needed both at local and national levels. A group of health professionals together with the consumer is a powerful influence to press health promotional activities. For instance, if the practice is in an inner city area with high unemployment and audit demonstrates that the majority of the population are overweight, undertake very little exercise and eat an inappropriate diet then a group of health professionals together with the community have the potential for pressing for leisure facilities.

The process of health promotion within Tannahill's framework reminds the nurse in general practice that as well as being accountable to ensure that one has competence in the relevant skills, one cannot work in isolation but has a distinct part to play in health promotional activity although not necessarily the total activity. The broad framework for health promotion can be applied to nursing in general practice, assisting the nurse to decide within that context, and within the context of other health professionals working in primary care, where her actual and potential role is or can be developed.

5.7 Health promotion in practice: the health professional's perspective

It is essential for the nurse in general practice to be able to consider her contribution to health promotion within the practice population and to be able to justify what that position is and evaluate specific health promotional activities. A framework on which to base her practice could be the Health Belief model, which is influenced by motivational theories and is particularly concerned with assessing factors that encourage compliance. It can be used to evaluate care to some extent.

Elements and cues are predicted assisting the nurse to gain the initial motivation of the patient to comply with health promotion initiatives. The Health Belief model is built on the following essentials:

● The individual's subjective state of readiness to take action in relation to their perception of susceptibility to an illness or the consequences of a particular illness.
● The individual's evaluation of the advocated health behaviour – i.e. its feasibility in relation to such things as physical and psychological 'barriers', age, sex, peer and reference groups.
● A 'cue' to action must occur to trigger the appropriate behaviour. This may be external or internal, for example, advice from another person or influence through the media (Becker and Maiman, 1975).

Table 5.1 illustrates this framework applied to a patient with non-insulin-dependent diabetes.

Table 5.1 Application of Health Belief model to a person with diabetes (non-insulin-dependent).

Individual perceptions	Modifying factors	Likelihood of action
	Life style impulsive Irregular working hours Perceived failure of other's treatment Love of 'sweet' food	Benefits Convenience of clinic times Seeing the same health professionals Adaptation of diabetes to life style
Knowledge of 'ill' diabetes and therefore severe illness *v.* not perceived as important because not on insulin	Perceived understanding of diabetes	Long term benefits Regular health checks Likelihood of compliance
	Educational input with leaflets, etc. Understanding need for checks as a preventive activity Family pressure	Barriers Diabetes = illness Inconvenient clinic times Seeing different people at clinic Waiting times Diet/medication Weight

This approach, as well as acknowledging the importance of the individual's perceptions, also considers external factors that influence the uptake of care. It emphasises the subjective state of the individual but does not include the dimension of personal and socio-cultural perceptions associated with symptoms, disease and health. With further development the framework could be useful in applying an approach to health education to increase the motivation of the patient to understand the benefits of changing health behaviour (Davidhazar, 1983). Health promotion is about helping people to adapt a change in health behaviour to their lifestyle. The framework also indicates a means of assessing factors that influence compliance.

As has been argued previously, health promotion is not an activity that can be undertaken by an individual. It is an activity that encompasses not only health professionals but whole communities with their infrastructure.

By identifying both a contextual and an individual framework, nursing in general practice is able to justify and present a role in health promotion in spite of limitations of the GP Contract. Indeed, by using a framework, there is a greater opportunity to be proactive and challenge health promotional activities within general practice.

5.8 Health promotion in practice: the patient's perspective

There are ethical and moral issues concerned with health promotional activity. The danger of attracting people, who previously considered themselves to be healthy, into clinics and telling them they are not as healthy as they thought they were has been highlighted (McBean, 1992). Other factors to be considered must include the aim for the health promotion activity – whether it has a cosmetic effect or a realistic outcome. The screening process may harm few people but the subsequent treatment could be damaging to more people as well as anxiety provoking.

Heart attacks and strokes also occur within a large group of people with a normotensive blood pressure reading. The Oxford and Collaborators Health Check trial (Oxcheck), funded by Imperial Cancer Research, is an ambitious study commencing in 1992. It is planned to sustain follow-up on patients for at least 3 years and is based on five general practices. The study aims to assess the effectiveness of nurse administered health checks in reducing: 'the prevalence of tobacco smoking, the mean section cholesterol, blood pressure and body mass index in a general practice population' (O'Neill, 1992). One of the seven subsidiary objectives is to 'explore the relationship between social factors, health beliefs and changes in behaviour'. The study hopes to dispel some of the concerns and confusion underpinning health promotion in general practice.

A person's optimum state of health has been defined as equivalent 'to the state of a set of conditions which fulfil and enable a person to work to fulfil his or her realistic chosen and biological potentials' (Seedhouse, 1988).

A further moral dimension can be included because of the possible need to prioritise either the 'cure' of the potential disease or the personal liberty of choice. If these are in conflict, then there is an urgent need to find a way to resolve these issues. There is, therefore, an increasingly ethical component in the area of health promotion. It is a question of deliberating about which health interventions are morally justified and to respect the rights of people to make choices and maintain their autonomy. This returns to the significance of clinical reasoning and professional judgement. These issues are likely to become part of the priorities in health promotion activities (Seedhouse, 1986).

5.9 Resources for planning health promotion activities

Health promotion may be seen as generating income for the practice and have arguably only a minimal impact on the practice population. The growing influence on the FHSA to develop service agreements with the GP provider units to target particular health promotional activities and the changes from July 1993 will result in a more strategic approach. Factors that influence what these should be include:

● Practice profiles.
● Locality health profiles.
● Consumer perceived needs.
● Prescribing patterns.
● Public health data.

FHSA's corporate contracts with the Regional Health Authority also include health promotional activities and are negotiated with the influence of health data on a regional and local level. Health Promotion Units are also influential in providing resources and training. Perhaps the major criticism for nursing in general practice has been the lack of preparation for running the clinics.

Unpublished data from two FHSAs in 1992 indicate that although nurses in general practice were running the majority of the clinics, about half of these clinics were being run by nurses with no additional preparation apart from a basic nursing qualification. Concern is expressed by nurses themselves. However, the main concerns are about professional competence and the perceived task oriented approach to health promotion by the employing GP. Aspects of skill mix have previously been addressed in Chapter 3 and in more detail in Chapter 6 and can be applied in this context. It is evident that in some practices, helpers undertake some of the data collection such as height, weight and urinalysis. However, learning needs are gradually being addressed and GPs are being asked to identify the qualifications of those running the clinics. Facilitators in collaboration with Family Health Services Authorities, GPs and Health Promotion Units play an important role in this process. A number of 'in house' educational programmes have been developed which are specifically targeted around health promotional activities. Nurses in general practice have a potential and actual role but need to be clear of this role within the total context of health promotion and to access resources to enable effective outcomes for health.

Whatever the specific area and aim, health promotion cannot be seen in isolation. Nursing in general practice may need to address this issue and ensure that health promotion is an activity shared by all health professionals and those with responsibility for the community environment, all of whom aim to empower the individual, the group and the community to make informed choices about health issues.

Summary

Health promotion is one of the key developments in general practice and has been influential in confirming nursing in general practice. It is also the potential base on which to move towards more collaboration with other agencies to enhance the opportunities of equality in health choices. In the context of the three main areas of health education, prevention and screening, the nurse in general practice has the potential to be proactive in making contributions that influence both the individual and the practice population.

There is also the responsibility to ensure that the patient is free to make informed health choices. Evaluation and audit is an integral part of professional accountability and the nurse in general practice will need to reflect how this is most effectively achieved in order to offer quality standards of practice for patient care.

References

Becker M and Maiman L (1975), Sociobehavioural determinants of compliance with health and medical care recommendations. *Medical Care*, **XIII** (1), pp. 10–21.

Cumberlege J (1986), *Report of the Community Nursing Review 'Neighbourhood Nursing – A Focus for Care'*. London: HMSO.

Damant M (1990), *Report of the Review Group for the Education and Training for Practice Nursing 'The Challenges of Primary Health Care in the 1990s'*. London: (ENB).

Davidhazar R (1983), Critique of the health-belief model. *Journal of Advanced Nursing*, **8**(6), pp. 467–472.

DOH (1987), *Promoting Better Health*. London: DOH.

DOH (1989), *Working for Patients*. Working paper 6. London: HMSO.

DOH (1992), *The Health of the Nation – a Summary of the Strategy for Health in England*. London: HMSO.

DOH Nursing Division (1989), *A Strategy for Nursing*. London: HMSO.

DHSS (1986b) *Primary Health Care – an Agenda for Discussion*. London: HMSO.

Donabedian A (1989), Institutional and professional responsibilities in quality assurance. *Quality Assurance Health Care*, **1**, pp. 3–11.

Griffiths J (1990), A new GP contract for health promotion? *Primary Health Care Management*, **1** (1), pp. 8–10.

McBean S F (1992), Promoting positive health. *Primary Health Care*, **2** (4), pp. 10–14.

Mahler H (1979), What is health for all? *World Health*, **Nov**, pp. 2–5.

NHS Management Executive (1991), *Framework of Audit for Nursing Services*. NHSME.

NHS Management Executive (1992), *Health Promotion and the GP Contract – Proposals for Consultation with GMSC*. FHSL(92)36.

O'Neill C (1992), Understanding the Oxcheck trial. *Primary Health Care*, **2** (6), pp. 5–8.

Payne L (1983), Health: a basic concept in nursing theory. *Journal of Advanced Nursing*, **8** (5), pp. 393–395.

Reid P (1979), Health for all by the year 2000. *World Health*, **Nov**, pp. 22–24.

Royal College of Nursing (1991), *Standards of Care Practice Nursing*. RCN.

Royal College of Nursing (1992), *Issues in Nursing and Health – Approaches to Nursing Care*. B.RCN.

Seedhouse D (1988), *Ethics: the Heart of Health Care*. Chichester: Wiley.

Smail S (1990), Health promotion and the new GP contract. *Practice Nurse*, **Feb**, pp. 391–392.

Tannahill A. (1985), What is health promotion? *Health Educational Journal*, **44** (4), pp. 167–168.

UKCC (1986), *Project 2000: a New Preparation for Practice*. London: UKCC.

WHO (1978), Declaration of Alma Ata 'Health for all by the Year 2000'. Geneva: WHO.

6 Management issues

Management and research issues have been addressed within the same chapter because of the complementary nature of the two activities. For example, the management activity of audit can prompt questions about practice and the trade-off between quality and quantity.

The integration of both activities within everyday practice is a key element of professional accountability as the following standards suggest:

> Leadership and management must be seen as an integral part of the role of nurses, midwives and health visitors. They have a vital contribution to make to strategic and operational policy making; to manpower planning; to delivery.
>
> (Strategy 61 Leadership and management: Enabling the work to be done)

> All clinical practice should be founded on up-to-date information and research findings; practitioners should be encouraged to identify the needs and opportunity for research presented by their work. Academic faculties with departments of nursing should be encouraged to broaden their links with, and deepen their expertise in, research-based practice'. (Targets for Practice 8 and 9).
>
> (DOH Nursing Division,1989)

To demonstrate these standards this chapter recognises the relative freedom of nurses in general practice to lead and innovate. The constraints under which they work are also taken into account, for example the time factor and pressure of appointment systems, and often the lack of support and adequate safeguards.

The employment relationship between GP and nurse is explored in some detail because of the value which nurses in general practice have always placed on this arrangement. Secondly, the climate of change in the NHS will present nurses with a range of contractual opportunities which need to be properly understood and negotiated. Thirdly, the issue of skill mix and paperless record systems is examined in relation to the implications for professional accountability, management and research.

It is not the intention of this chapter to replicate the material available in the many useful textbooks on management and research, rather to broaden the reader's thinking, raise questions about current practice and stimulate further enquiry.

6.1 Management challenges and resources

Clearly the complementary problem solving processes of management and research provide an integrating framework for all the processes which were seen to characterise nursing in general practice in Chapter 1. The important contribution of this branch of community nursing to the health of the nation is reinforced by Virginia Bottomley's endorsement of the Roy Report 'Nursing in the Community' (1991) in which she stated:

> For most of us, the community and family health services are the main point of contact within the NHS. We must not underestimate the impact of the services provided in the community or general practice setting, nor the contribution nurses make to the delivery of these services.

The working group chaired by Sheila Roy was commissioned by the NHS Management Executive to 'consider the management principles which should inform the purchasing, organisation and provision of nursing services in the community in the light of opportunities by the Government's three white papers, i.e. *Promoting Better Health* (DOH, 1987); *Working for Patients* (DOH, 1989); and *Caring for People* (DOH, 1989)'. The key management principles identified by the working group have already been addressed in previous chapters but to recap, these principles are:

● A shared vision of care.
● A commitment to joint working and putting patients first.
● The joint assessment of population health needs.
● Joint strategies which clearly set out the responsibility of each agency.
● Effective communications.
● A commitment to quality as a key management principle.

The relationship between these principles and the processes which underpin nursing in general practice is crucial to the development of the profession and the outcome of the care provided. The combination of the two provides the foundation for a systematic approach to integrated services in the community which cooperate with hospital-based services. Furthermore, it offers a framework for the integration of the wide range of nursing expertise currently available in the community. It is a framework which could provide a springboard for change and the implementation of any proposals made for nursing in the community. In addition, the challenge of social policy will embrace the core skills and discipline of management as an enabling process and research as a systematic approach to developing practice.

Enabling is a central concept of management, whether applied to the management of patient care, staff or the organisation. **Figure 6.1** presents a summary of some key management processes.

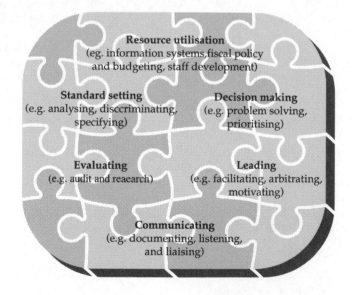

Figure 6.1 Key management processes.

Nurses in general practice are moving forward as part of a complex and sophisticated branch of health care. New systems and organisational structures will be introduced which require him/her to play a full and active part in the cost effective management of health care and to validate the nursing contribution. Perhaps one of the first questions to be asked is, what are the range of nursing skills required in general practice ?

6.1.1 Skill mix

Skill (and grade) mix is usually defined as:

> the balance between trained staff and untrained, qualified and unqualified, and supervisory and operative staff within a service area as well as different staff groups. The optimum skill mix is achieved when a desired standard of service is provided at the minimum cost, which is consistent with the efficient deployment of trained, qualified and supervisory personnel and the maximisation of contributions from all staff ... Grade mix is one component of a wider skill mix exercise which looks at the numbers of qualified nursing staff required of certain grades.
>
> (RCN, 1992)

Skill mix has its roots in the industrial division of labour model of management. Lizbeth Hockey was one of the first researchers to examine the relevance of this approach to nursing outside the hospital setting. Her studies explored this concept in relation to differently qualified members of staff within District Nursing teams. Hockey's research identified the relative merits of a team approach in which the diversity of nursing skill reflected the needs of a given population (Hockey 1966, 1968 and 1972). The next set of substantive data to emerge resulted from the Review of Nursing Skill Mix (DOH, 1986). The Review was described as 'a reconnaissance into territory that has never been comprehensively mapped out'. Although the study sample was drawn from the hospital setting, the findings establish some useful principles for nurses involved in a similar exercise in general practice settings. For instance the Report states that:

> Training, management, financial and analytical support should be provided to facilitate the effective operation of ward sisters and charge nurses so that they can:
> – use a systematic approach to assess the needs of their patients and how they can be met;
> – make the best use of information in determining the skill mix, level and effective utlisation of nursing staff;
> – contribute to management budgeting in the pursuit of delivery of a cost-effective service.

Reflecting upon the seemingly arbitrary way in which non-nursing duties have been determined and assigned to persons whose names do not appear on the Professional Register maintained by UKCC, the Report makes encouraging reading. A typical example of such arbitrary decisions of the past were those relating to the nutritional needs of patients, e.g. selecting from a menu, serving and supervising the meal was designated as a non-nursing duty in the face of evidence which indicated that some patients leave hospital malnourished and dehydrated (e.g. Smith, 1972). This is a startling realisation considering the importance of nutrition in the promotion of health and healing. An excellent observation which is made from time to time is that there is nothing basic about basic nursing (MacFarlane, 1970).

Nurses in general practice need to give careful consideration to the introduction of skill mix. On the one hand, there is the danger that indiscriminate decisions could be made in the absence of the education, skill and resources recommended in the DOH Skill Mix Review quoted above. On the other hand, opportunities could be lost if the appropriate steps are not taken to ensure that optimum use is made of the professional role of the nurse in general practice. The designation of practice nurse has been defined as follows:

> A practice nurse should hold an appropriate qualification which is registered or recorded on the effective part of the Professional Register maintained by the United Kingdom Central Council (UKCC). This will normally be a Registered General Nurse. Where activities are undertaken for which a specific qualification is required, for instance health visiting, midwifery or district nursing, the person will be expected to hold the appropriate qualification of Registered Health Visitor, Registered Midwife or a recordable qualification in District Nursing. Where the practice nurse holds the qualification of Enrolled Nurse (General) only and is on Parts 2 or 7 of the UKCC Professional Register, then he or she may only undertake a limited range of duties, having due regard to the skills of enrolled nurses contained within the nurse training Rules of the UKCC. In addition, the Registered Midwife must be a practising midwife as defined in the UKCC Midwives Rules.
>
> (DOH and Welsh Office, 1990)

Clearly, perhaps unwittingly, there has been a lack of understanding of the Rules laid down by UKCC and much concern has been expressed about the vulnerability of the nurse, her/his employer and the patients for whom care is provided (Damant, 1990).

Nurses in the UK are not alone in their awareness of the potential dangers; some nurses in the USA are also expressing concern about the deleterious effect of 'undiscriminated nursing practice' on health care. Whilst the situation in the USA is not directly comparable with that of the UK, in principle, we share the same concern for a systematic approach to differentiated practice and skill mix in order to:

● Secure the highest possible standard of nursing care for the individual, the family and the community.
● Preserve the integrity of the professional role of the nurse whilst maximising alternative resources in the face of the increasing complexity and rising costs of health care (Briggs, 1982).

It is interesting to note that the same principle is implicit within the Strategy for Nursing and RCN guidance on skill mix and reprofiling. Another American

Study referred to in the DOH Skill Mix Review concludes that the 'rate of omissions in nursing care is inversely related to the level of education, skill and experience of the practitioner' (Miller and Bryant, 1965).

For nursing in general practice, it is timely to consider such findings. The ENB Review found that practice nursing may not be the exclusive preserve of the registered general nurse (RGN), although the finding was based an a rather incomplete data base (Damant, 1990). Enrolled nurses, children's nurses (RCN) and nurses for the mentally ill (RNMI) sought clarification from the Department, the UKCC and their professional associations about their position within general practice and their professional accountability. The Department responded by including the definition of practice nurse within the Statement of Fees and Allowances payable to General Medical Practitioners of England and Wales. Guidance was also given by the statutory body concerning their professional accountability in a Statement on Practice Nurses and Aspects of the new GP Contract (UKCC, 1990).

If the nursing needs of a local community are to be appropriately served, a range of nursing expertise can be cost-effectively deployed within the nursing team in general practice. But an important part of the skill mix exercise is to take into account the wide variation in the social and occupational characteristics of practice nurses identified by several studies (Reedy *et al.*, 1976; Greenfield *et al.*, 1987). Occupational traits and professional values seem to range from those consistent with an autonomous practitioner of nursing to the narrow reductionist model of care dictated by doctor delegated tasks aimed to relieve the doctor's workload and inspired by the 'doctor knows best' mentality. To quote from the evidence submitted by individual practice nurses as part of the ENB Review (Damant, 1990). Practice nurses:

- need to be good RGNs with a lot of common sense (the need for additional training was not necessarily an important factor);
- are a group of nurses who enjoy their work and the time arrangement which fits in with personal commitments;
- generally do not have the time to undertake a demanding training;
- are completely separate and different from other spheres of nursing, the obligation of the practice nurse being to the doctor rather than to other members of the PHCT.

(Para 4.2.2, Message No. 1)

At the other end of the spectrum, evidence supported the wider concept of professional autonomy and teamwork which reflected an individualised holistic approach to care. To quote:

- Practice nurses who are health visitors use all their health visiting skills in a very rewarding and useful way;
- the future training of practice nurses should develop along academic as well as along practical lines;
- we are fully committed to the concept that learning together enables people to work together; it is imperative to retain the course in higher education for the breadth and scope of the learning process.

(Para 4.2.2, Message No.2)

Clearly the development of practice nursing is at a watershed when to draw rigid divisions of labour might stifle initiative and growth, but on the other hand not to consider the implications of different abilities, motivation and levels of clinical reasoning could equally result in the dilution of professional skills and quality care.

Is there a case for a nursing skill mix in general practice? Is there a place for differently qualified nurses and support workers in the general practice nursing team? Is the example discussed in Chapter 3 a way forward for the future? How are nurses to be encouraged and prepared to push out the traditional frontiers of the role into specialised areas of practice in order to extend the range of nursing care available to the individual, the family and the community, and to provide a consultancy service for their peers and other members of the health and social services team? These issues are discussed and signposted in the Strategy for Nursing, Targets 16 and 17 and in the Department's view of the extending role of the nurse (PL/CMO (89)7 PL/CNO (89)10 and HC(77)22). The Department's view is that:

> the role of the nurse is continually developing as changes in practice and training add new functions to the normal range of duties ... No profession whose functions are as diverse as nursing can maintain or improve standards of health care and be flexible enough to meet continually changing demands unless continuous attention is given to education and to the planning and evaluation of experimental studies designed to improve nursing practices ... extending the role of the nurse remains crucial to the provision and development of patient care.

The professional and legal implications of such developments are set out in (HC(77)22 para 3), the Code of Professional Conduct for the Nurse, Midwife and Health Visitor (UKCC, 1992a) and the Scope of Professional Practice (UKCC, 1992b). With these views in mind it will be interesting to observe the progress and outcomes of the 22 nurse practitioner experimental studies currently in progress in the South East Thames Region. This will give a new dimension to skill mix and develop the work pioneered by Stilwell (1982).

Clearly the notion of skill mix has developed beyond the traditional boundaries of the past; nevertheless there still remain some possible advantages and disadvantages which need to be considered in relation to today's notion of 'skill mix'. For example, the advantages are seen to include:

- The cost effective use of resources.
- Enhanced quality of care and job satisfaction.
- Improved consumer satisfaction.

The disadvantages to be safeguarded against may still include:

- Fragmentation, boredom and repetition.
- A hierarchy which is devaluing and results in the loss of self esteem.
- Expediency, i.e. the cheapest commodity rather than the 'best buy'.
- Vulnerability /security of tenure and deskilling.

(Hoffman and Wyly, 1979; Hockey, 1972).

The processes involved in assessing the skill mix required in a particular general practice setting or locality are complex. One such process is first to assess the health care needs and the general practice population's need for nursing as the basis for job design, or role specification, prior to making decisions about the grading and the skill mix needs of the practice. It is now intended to consider some of the issues related to health need assessment and job design, or role specification.

6.2 The analysis of health care needs

The assessment of need and the identification of those needs which can best be met by nursing as a composite part of a multiprofessional whole is a complex process.

Firstly, this predisposes a clear understanding of the role definition and function of nursing. Chapters 2 and 3 considered the essence of nursing in relation to the ways in which clinical practice might be defined and standards improved. The central themes of the debate were:

● The relationship between nursing and medicine.
● The characteristics of nursing as a specific discipline directed towards assisting people with actual/potential health needs which have the propensity to interrupt their daily lives.
● Patient advocacy and empowerment.

Secondly, it presupposes a comprehensive, accurate and up-to-date data base. It is doubtful whether the clinical audit approach in itself can provide the scope and flexibility for targeting the practice population's nursing need. Epidemiology, in isolation to demographic information of local and national populations, fails to reflect some of the human elements associated with morbidity and mortality. Roy stressed the value of a 'bottom-up' approach in which the practitioner has a key role, in partnership with the patient, and within the broad context of multiprofessional practice for the 'joint assessment of population needs'. The RCN extends the parameters of the debate by encouraging nurses to recognise the importance of working with their managers in deciding how best nurses can be deployed (RCN, 1992). Clearly, the assessment of health needs and the implication for nursing in general practice is a multifactorial activity which includes the professionals and consumers working in partnership (Wilkin *et al.*, 1992).

Various strategies are being developed and it is very necessary that nurses in general practice are up-to-date and familiar with the approach taken by the Family Health Services Authority, or within their own practice. Nurses also need to develop an awareness of Social Policy and to have access to guidelines issued by the Department of Health and the professional bodies in this regard. Reading and 'keeping an ear to the ground' are essential skills in present day practice. The rapidly changing scene makes it inappropriate to offer more detailed guidelines for managing this difficult area of change and safeguarding patient care. Suffice it to add that nurses in general practice will need to examine and evaluate the various formulae and frameworks produced for the purpose of analysing and assessing health care needs in the light of the previous chapters and to consider whether there are more appropriate approaches. For instance, some nurse theorists have produced several useful frameworks from which to choose.

Traditionally, America has led the field in developing models and theories of nursing practice which can be used as an analytical and evaluative tool. For example, Neuman's System Theory offers a holistic perspective of the patient, or patient populations, and a means of assessing the positive and negative forces for health and the indicators for nursing (Neuman, 1980). Neuman's work has been widely adapted for this purpose in various spheres of clinical practice, management and education. Its adaptation for the assessment of community health needs is well documented. (Neuman, 1982; Anderson *et al.*, 1986).

Whichever model or framework is used for the purpose of assessing the health needs of the community, it is critical for the outcome that the formula and process are able to accommodate health as the complex phenomenon and dynamic concept of 'wholeness' described in previous chapters. A formula is needed which identifies not only need but also the resources available/required to address such needs. It is important to remember that resources lie within individuals, their kinship networks and wider social context, as well as the public, private and voluntary sector provisions.

Clearly, a comprehensive assessment relies upon a mulitprofessional, teamworking approach which includes the consumer. Because of the fragmented nature of nursing in the community, it will be essential to adopt a strategy which captures and integrates the different offerings and expertise for the ultimate benefit of the patient/client and the effective utilisation of skilled resources.

Community nursing in the generic sense has a responsibility to recognise and accept its collective accountability to society for ensuring that the health needs of both stable and unstable communities are systematically assessed, and that nursing as a resource for health is identified.

For some groups of clients, particularly those who require complex or expensive packages of services, it is envisaged that a care management function in conjunction with social services will be introduced. PHCTs are expected to contribute to the collaborative process and further improve liaison between agencies (Audit Commission, 1992).

A reduction in the present socioeconomic differences which produce inequalities in health are a priority for all disciplines – the health and welfare professions, spiritual leaders, and the secular community. However difficult and challenging, the rigour of a systematic approach to the assessment of health needs is axiomatic.

Assessment of the health needs of a community/nation provides an important basis from which to plan both service *and education* strategies – education and training are essential resources. UKCC acknowledged the difficulty of the task which formed part of the Project 2000 (UKCC, 1986). The profession now awaits the results of the second stage of this comprehensive review – the post-registration education and practice project (PREPP). The challenge will be to achieve a process of reconciliation that will override the limitations imposed by the traditional boundaries within community nursing, thereby offering a more holistic and integrated position for future learners and practitioners to enjoy. In this regard, the Audit Commission recognises the vital importance of a shift from the historical position which promoted the profession to that of the primacy of the patient/client and the health of the nation.

The demands for a systematic, comprehensive assessment of health needs constitute an argument for multiprofessional education through which core skills and practices can be developed and collective (and individual) accountability enhanced. Furthermore, it is central to decisions concerning skill mix.

The next step will be to identify and design an appropriate role/job specification of people working within the practice.

6.3 'Job' design

The job design should spell out the functions and responsibilities associated with the specific role of the practitioner within the practice. It involves the process of identifying the job content, the methods and processes to be used; the relationships within and between organisations and the resources required (Armstrong, 1988). A 'job' is suggested to have two main aims:

● To satisfy the requirements of the organisation (which in this context includes the consumer and wider community) in terms of productivity, efficiency and quality.
● To satisfy the needs of the individual (in this context the practitioner) for interest, challenge and accomplishment.

Job design is a process which is closely related to grading and the level of remuneration, and therefore it has implications for the employment contract discussed later in the chapter.

The outcome of the job design may be a job description or a role specification depending upon the style of management and the requirements of the practice in terms of nursing.

The difference between job description and role specification is quite important in terms of a conceptual framework. The two terms are not totally interchangeable, although they both relate to the contract between the employer, or contractor and the employee, or sub-contractor. It is likely that the transition from practice nursing to nursing in general practice will best be facilitated by the latter approach. The job description is less likely to offer the desired flexibility and potential for creative practice and the exercise of professional autonomy. With these observations in mind, the job design framework will be used to demonstrate the essential features of a contractual arrangement.

The 'tools' required to complete these processes are many and various. A formal Work Study may be conducted. On the other hand, an in-house activity may be undertaken based on the systematic observation of practice and diary analysis. This may involve peer review, or a self-reflective process using critical incidences, noting that in this context the judgement focuses on the incident and not the practitioner. Task analysis could also, with caution, form part of the activity, bearing in mind that when set within the context of comprehensive care, the most seemingly simple psychomotor task may involve complex cognitive processes.

The evaluation of the job design/specification and its ability to meet the declared aims is essential. The complementary processes of clinical audit, appraisal and performance review could contribute to the evaluation by assessing the extent to which the potential of the job has been realised and/or constrained.

Of prime importance is the level of expertise in terms of the skills, knowledge and resources required to manage this process, to use the tools to their full potential, evaluate and where necessary change or modify them. For nurses in general practice, this important issue will be discussed later in relation to the contract of service and its management. Of equal importance is the standard, kind and content of the documentation of nursing care provided in the practice, and its accessibility. There are two aspects to be considered. One refers to previous references to the assessment of health care needs and includes a composite *practice data base*, e.g. age, sex register and records/protocols for interventions within and between organisations are critical factors. In many instances this information will be summarised in, or augmented by the *practice report* (Pringle, 1990). In addition, many FHSAs are preparing the *locality health profile* in collaboration with the Public Health Department and Health Authority; this will be a valuable resource for planners and practitioners of health care. The second aspect is the specific *record of nursing care* which is now considered at some length.

6.4 Nursing care records in general practice

This documentation is an account of the treatment and care delivered by nurses in the health centre, clinic or surgery. These records can be used for many purposes. Clearly all records are an essential part of the process of identifying and evaluating the unique role of the nurse in general practice. We are rapidly approaching a paperless system of record keeping which has been the result of many years of innovation, refinement and change. Leicester City Health Department's computerisation of District Nursing records was one of the early pioneers in the field (Eccles, 1977). Since this time numerous schemes have been developed, some even anticipating the advent of the European Community; the Exmouth Health Care Card Scheme is giving an international lead in such developments (Hall and Hopkins, 1990; Hopkins, 1990). It is therefore timely to ask in this climate of value for money, what records do nurses in general keep and what records should they keep? Do existing records provide a basis for skills analysis and 'job' design? To what extent do the records ensure a safe, acceptable, accessible, service with due regard to confidentiality and the accountability of the nurse? There could be many ways of examining these issues but perhaps the critical test might be to ask whether the records document what might be seen as the five central elements of nursing, namely:

● Care that is safe, has continuity (including shared care) for the individual/family/community which is accessible, acceptable and affordable (WHO, 1978).
● Leadership/management which provides protection for the practitioner, his/her employers/peers and colleagues within and between agencies. Will the records assist the management processes referred to in **Figure 6.1**?
● Enquiry and research whereby the records offer a valuable resource of systematically obtained information about nursing in general practice. What do nurses in general practice do? Are there different types and approaches to nursing in practice? The ENB review would suggest that there are. Are there differences in the levels of clinical reasoning? The point has been made in

Chapter 2 that we need to know more about these differences. Clearly, in order to answer these and many other such questions, documented evidence of all kinds is crucial.

● Teaching and facilitating. Health records are a rich source of discovery learning. One approach examines the value of 'The Baliant Random Case Analysis' for peer assessment and as a teaching (preferably multidisciplinary) method for students of health care (Buckley, 1990). The concept of critical incident analysis as part of the process of professional and personal development and the Assessment of Prior Experiential Learning (APEL), also requires access to a comprehensive record system (Welsh National Board for Nursing, Midwifery and Health Visiting, 1991; RCN, 1991).The focus is the learning which has taken place in the course of practice.

● Member of a profession. It is through the documentation of practice that the values and beliefs of the profession are articulated, evaluated and questioned. Nursing records are an instrument of the practitioner's accountabilty to the society he/she serves and represent the extent of the practitioner's responsibility to safeguard the patient/client against unsound practice through acts of ommission or commission. Quality assurance is implicit within the Code of Professional Conduct and the Scope of Professional Practice for the Nurse, Midwife and Health Visitor (UKCC,1992a and b). A clear and sensitive use of the case study approach to demonstrate the practitioner's accountability for the quality of care and the standard of professional conduct expected of the Registered Nurse has been produced to guide the practitioner and to stimulate discussion with peers, employers and management (Pyne, 1992). Not all case studies are directly related to community care setting but in asking 'Could this happen where you work?'; Pyne isolates two essential principles of professional accountability, namely the obligation to provide reasonable care, and to uphold the integrity of the profession.

To summarise, nursing records are an important resource which contributes to cost effective, quality care in general practice. For the purpose of job analysis and the determination of skill mix they are an essential tool. They can contain information, documenting patient care, assisting the management function, producing data for investigation and research and providing a legal safeguard for the patient, the nurse and the employer.

The next logical step is to consider the Contract of Service.

6.5 Contracts of service

The purchaser/provider roles directing future organisations, systems of health care and management strategies will result in an experience for both the consumer and practitioner that is vastly different to the traditional approach (Audit Commission, 1992). The 'old system' which, by comparison, was generally less cost conscious and perhaps less responsive to change is replaced by competition and the assumption of increased responsiveness and efficiency. This will have far reaching effects. As a consequence, several questions emerge which will need to be addressed in detail if the full implications and opportunities of a revitalised health service are to be grasped by the profession. The professional organisations and trade unions are making available the expertise, advice and guidance to members. At the outset of a new, value for money, era of health care it is thought provoking to consider such issues as 'Is the nurse in general practice purchaser or provider – might she/he be both?'; 'How might the 'employment' status of practice nurses be affected ?'

The security and safety aspects of employment and the factors which distinguish the 'employee' from the 'contractor' need to be fully understood and carefully considered (Whincup, 1982). For instance, nurses in general practice are currently employees of an individual general practitioner, or company, i.e. the practice/group of general practitioners. Might the future provide opportunities for 'partnerships', or 'independent/self employed contracts'? What will be the implications of such contractual arrangements (Ham, 1990; Dixon, 1990)? Numerous expert texts are regularly produced giving guidance on employment law and regulations, trade union facilities, and the protection and activities offered by the professional associations.

Whincup's material is summarised in **Figure 6.2** as a diagrammatic illustration of the contractual framework in terms of:

● What the law requires (conditions of service).
● Personal agreements between the contractor and the contractee (role specification).

For current regulations reference should be made to Department of Employment Guidelines (PL 700 and PL 919).

The legal framework within nursing can be regarded as having two main elements. General law, of which employment law is a good example and the

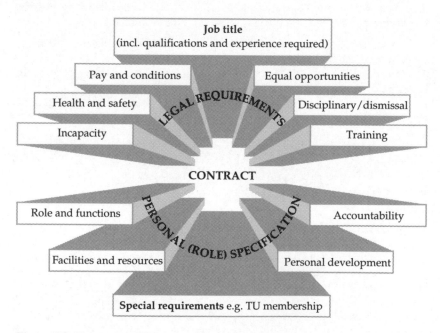

Figure 6.2 The contractual framework.

statutory regulations through which the profession of nursing is empowered and controlled (Nurses, Midwives and Health Visitors Act, 1978 and 1992). The Code of Professional Conduct for the Nurse, Midwife and Health Visitor (UKCC, 1992a) and The Scope of Professional Practice for the Nurse, Midwife and Health Visitor (UKCC, 1992b) are statements which describe the behaviour to be expected of the registered practitioner, it also provides the nurse, midwife or health visitor with a negotiating tool for improvements in health care. There are of course occasions where the nurse's behaviour may be seen to have contravened the laws of the country, and/or to have infringed the statutory standards laid down by the profession, e.g. assault, misappropriation of another's property, the misuse of harmful substances.

Within the new organisations and systems of health care and welfare, nurses in general practice will need to develop a greater awareness of the legal framework within which they practice and to use it as a resource for better patient care rather than as a negative constraining force. The contractual framework within which the nurse functions will be an important vehicle towards these goals. For instance, if the practitioner is self employed, he/she rather than the employer will need to take into account the contractual legal requirements. If, however, the practice nurse is an independent practitioner, similar to the 'independent midwife' for example, she/he may be a purchaser of other professional services for her/his patients, client group – yes, even medical care!

In conclusion, what is it, in terms of the service contract, that the employee needs from the organisational structure in general practice? **Figure 6.3** sets out the three central strands. In large organisations these strands represent separate functions with a discrete set of skills and knowledge. However, in general practice these functions may be amalgamated and assigned to one person, usually the GP or the practice manager. The value and importance of these functions should not be underestimated; it is essential that nurses in general practice have access to expert advice, counsel, information and support in all of these spheres. The amalgamation of these functions can create role conflict for the post holder. For example, personnel services can bridge difficulties and arbitrate for the employee on administrative and professional issues. Likewise, the professional practice manager has proved to be a necessary asset where

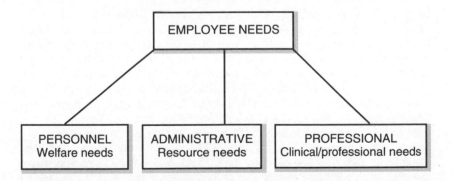

Figure 6.3 The contract of employment – the needs of the employee.

general practice has increased in size and complexity because he/she will be in a position to identify and meet the needs of the professional clinicians and show respect for their expertise. For instance, the management of the treatment room is part of the professional nurse's accountability to the patient to ensure a safe environment. The scope of nursing in general practice and the range of interventions from the 'simple' to the 'complex' has been widely acknowledged (Bowlden and Tackle, 1989). In addition, the nurse is professionally responsible for the upkeep of equipment and knowledge about its correct usage, including the disposal of waste (Jeffree, 1990). Jeffree also considers the value of the nurse's involvement in the planning of the treatment room because of her understanding of the application of ergonomic principles in the caring environment and the requirements of Health and Safety at Work legislation in the clinical setting. The nurse's responsibility in this regard will expand as the recommendations of the Working Group on Nurse Prescribing (DOH Nursing Division, 1990) are introduced.

It is inevitable that situations will arise which are complex and delicate and where expert professional advice is required by the nurse who, unlike people employed in other ways, may not have direct access to this resource. In such situations the needs of the nurse in general practice can be provided for through a number of channels, for example many FHSAs employ Nurse Advisers. Medicine and nursing are separate professional entities and whilst they may share the same professional ethic and commitment to clinical practice, and to some extent their skills and knowledge base may be seen to overlap, each is personally accountable for the quality of care provided within the practice, as it relates to the standards and expectations of their specific profession. There are also many other anomalies in general practice which increase the nurse's need for professional support and guidance; for example the nurse's role in a dispensing practice may include the dispensing of multiple doses of drug substances for self administration. One might argue that, in principle, this is not significantly different from the administration/prescribing of a single dose/application. Is it, and does it matter who dispenses? It would appear to be more appropriate to delegate dispensing duties to the nurse who is able to give accurate information and health education, rather than to the receptionist who would be less well informed. In such circumstances there are two critical questions to which the nurse must respond.

Firstly, is she/he competent and does she/he feel confident in her competence to undertake this function? Secondly, does the activity contribute to comprehensive nursing care of the patient? There is much evidence to suggest that the advice given by nurses to patients on the self administration of drug substances tends to achieve a significantly higher level of compliance compared with situations where advice was given by the doctor (Ross, 1988, 1989). However, the final decision must be influenced by the extent to which this activity makes the best use of nursing skills and expertise within the practice and whether there are other aspects of health care which have a higher priority. The GP must ensure the competency of all persons to whom he delegates treatment and care within the practice, as required by the new GP Contract and the Complaints Procedure laid down by the FHSA. The key question which nurses must be in a position to answer and defend is 'How can nursing time within general practice be used to maximum effectiveness?'.

6.6 Performance review: process and benefits

The overriding component of good management is the appraisal, development and skilful deployment of human resources. The relative merit of appraisal and performance review is the contribution and rigour it brings to the assessment of quality – a process in which the nurse is expected to play a full and active part (Kerrane, 1989). Kerrane adopts the unequivocal stance that 'a good appraisal scheme will improve patient care at all levels by ensuring the personal and professional development of nurses'. But practitioners are often very wary and sceptical about the process and its outcome. How does such a scheme work, what will it achieve, is it relevant to my situation? These are some of the questions which are most often asked.

The short answer seems to be that the scheme will be as good and as effective as the participants want it to be. However, there are some stringent rules to be respected by both the appraiser and the appraisee. The whole process is based on mutual regard for each other's expertise and integrity. There are several useful training manuals and short courses to guide the person through the process which is generally regarded as something of a minefield. This section will briefly consider some of the features of appraisal and performance review in order that the nurse in general practice can think about it constructively. Briefly, the stages involve introduction and consultation about the scheme under consideration. Prior to the appraisal interview the appraisee is invited to assess their own performance, reflect on their accomplishments and difficulties. The appraisee is asked to consider whether the job fully utilises their skills, training, knowledge and interests – how might it be changed in order to be a more cost effective and positive experience.

Meanwhile, the appraiser is reflecting on the appraisee's performance, achievements and missed opportunities using both objective and subjective material. The job description may be evaluated against the needs of the service and the development of the appraisee. Likewise, the resources and support services provided by the employer will be examined and evaluated in relation to the appraisee's performance. The environment for the interview should be as carefully prepared as the participants. However, the important issues for nurses in general practice are, who will conduct the appraisal in which areas of practice, and what tools should be used? Kerrane stresses the importance of appraisal performance training. Since its inception in the 1970s performance review has had a close association with nursing audit and requires to be managed with the same skill and sensitivity (Wiseman, 1977). It is a process which demands respect and as such it is described as a tool which has no value until it is picked up and used towards some end, either constructively to build a house, or destructively to kill someone.

Performance review can result in some worthwhile achievements. It can be used as a two-way process of monitoring the 'Contract'. On the one hand, it seeks to assess whether or not the performance of the employee, or contractor is acceptable, i.e. is he/she meeting the agreed standard. On the other hand, it is a means of examining the extent to which the employer has fulfilled his/her obligations within the 'Contract' and provided the resources to do the job, e.g. training, equipment.

Clearly there is the potential for a conflict of values and priorities between the employee and employer. Is the standard expected by the employer the same as that towards which the employee is aiming? Examples of such conflicts have been experienced in relation to Health Promotion and Screening activities where productivity (quantity) is more highly valued than quality. At least the performance review should assist in the reconciliation of such conflicts, thus enabling a renegotiated position without compromising standards of care and the prioritising of professional time and accountability.

6.7 The management of time

Time, above all other resources at a professional's disposal, is the most critical. Time represents a whole galaxy of commodities which as part of a 'Contract' has a financial value. Yes, 'Time means money'. This will be amplified further in the final chapter as part of the general discussion on contractual agreements, rights and obligations. Meanwhile, the reader may wish to think about the cost of his/her own time and some of the problems associated with its management (Dingwall, 1983). Several other useful texts and exercises are available to guide you through the process. Dingwall issues a salutary reminder that *you* own your time, *you* make the decisions about how it is used, therefore it cannot be argued that someone else 'wasted' it for you. Readers may think this a bold statement to make in the light of the preceding discussion. You may well be asking how many patients can you see in 1 hour, and what is the trade-off between quality and quantity? Nurses in general practice will find the experience of their medical colleagues in the management of the consultation a useful approach to consider (Baliant and Norell, 1973). It is an approach which offers a constructive framework for the five elements of nursing outlined above in relation to record keeping. There are perhaps two questions which need to be asked in respect of the effective use of time, namely:

How and why do we prioritise our time in the way we do?

Nurses will need to address this issue in a systematic way by taking into account some of the following influences as part of problem solving:

● The frame of reference used to guide nursing practice will influence decisions about what is important and what is not. For example, an emphasis on the procedures in general practice may result in a high priority being given to 'the task', e.g. the venepuncture, whereas an emphasis on the context of care will lead to a more comprehensive and holistic approach. The latter is an approach which empowers the patient (The Patient's Charter; DOH, 1991) and creates a climate of care in which health education and clinical treatment are of equal importance. It is the foundation of a therapeutic alliance and mutual respect.
● Personal/professional aptitude, i.e. those things we know we are 'good at' and find rewarding, and which we might be tempted to do more often.
● Values. There is some evidence to suggest that nurses value some patients more than others (Stockwell, 1976). Stockwell suggests that in the hospital setting, the patients most disadvantaged were older people and the mentally ill and, as highlighted in Chapter 2, there might be differences in the treatment of some ethnic groups.

● Resources available, including the interest/collaboration of those with whom we work. Limited resources, management styles and negative attitudes can militate against the effective use of time, for example, an autocratic approach to the introduction of information technology, or the skills of a technician can result in them being perceived as a threat rather than a resource. Clearly the role of management is an important one in this regard.

● Lack of education and inadequate preparation in the management of time will be a handicap to those practitioners whose continuing education and training has not taken account of this increasingly important element of nursing practice and professional accountability.

The second question relates to the observation we have all made:

I don't know where today has gone.

Taking the old song 'There's a hole in my bucket dear Liza, dear Liza' as an analogy it may be an interesting and worthwhile exercise to complete the activity included in **Figure 6.4.** The purpose of the exercise is to encourage you to critically examine:

● The cause of your 'time leaks'.
● The ways in which you might 'plug' the leaks you have identified.

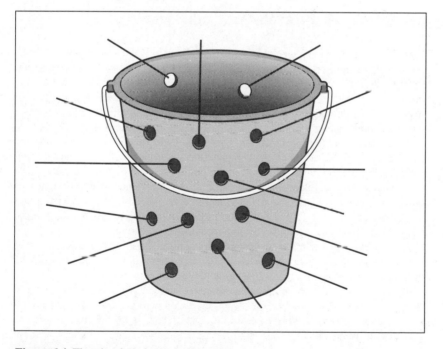

Figure 6.4 There's a hole in my bucket.

The process which has just been worked through could justifiably be regarded as an audit of clinical practice, i.e. the management of time. It is arguably the responsibility of every practitioner to ask such questions about their management of resources as part of their everyday routines, as well as being part of a more formalised process. Indeed Medical Audit in general practice has been a requirement since April 1991 in the belief that the systematic review of patient care is a key component of good practice (HC(FP)(90)8. Preparation for PHCTs is being arranged by some Departments of General Practice to facilitate attendance by the whole team, the GP, practice nurse and the practice manager, at the same time – another initiative for multiprofessional education. There is a widely held belief that 'audit of the organisation should not become another bureaucratic burden but a process of clinical enquiry that can enliven routine tasks and give prominence to previously neglected areas' (Buckley, 1990).

The results of such enquiries will inevitably challenge some aspects of current practice and point to the need for change based on a systematic assessment of the problem. Research is a tool which can assist this process. Nurses in general practice need to feel comfortable with the idea of questioning practice and become skilled in using research to achieve quality care and the effective use of resources. The final section of this chapter will now examine the value of research and the involvement of nurses in general practice.

6.8 Research: the systematic approach

This final section of Chapter 6 draws together the recurring belief that through the keeping of accurate records, the willingness and ability to share our successes and failures with others, the practice of nursing becomes more scientific and logical process. It is well documented that research in contemporary practice has an important role in rebutting the challenges from within and without at this time of unprecedented change (Bradshaw, 1989). Nursing in general practice is defined as a practice based discipline whose theory grows from and is tested in practice (Damant, 1990). Nurses need to recognise the ways in which they can question their practice and the value of so doing. Therefore nurses who play an active role as a teacher, or a facilitator of another's learning experience, need constantly to draw on research findings in order to aid the learner's ability to distil from and apply first principles to practice. Furthermore, Bradshaw argues that the teacher relies heavily on the research method to evaluate teaching systematically and identify the needs of learners. Nursing in general practice teaches a diverse population in different settings, therefore the assessment of learning needs and the evaluation of outcome is critical in a value for money economy.

It might be argued that research for nurses in general practice is a continuation of the systematic discipline which begins with a process versus a task orientation to care and problem solving in everyday practice. It is an approach which is extended to meet 'practice' goals in terms of protocols and packages of care, standard setting and clinical audit. Research and audit are sometimes seen to be separate activities but good audit projects can lead to small focused research questions (Buckley, 1990). Indeed, the Strategy for Nursing specifies the following justifications for the use of research findings in everyday practice:

● People are entitled to the best possible care. That care should be founded upon up-to-date sound information and scientific knowledge (Practice Target 7).
● Practitioners must foster a receptive attitude towards research, together with a commitment to pursue and apply it in the delivery of health care. Ensuring that the results of current research are effectively disseminated to all health care settings and promptly incorporated into standard treatments and procedures (para 22).

Research can be pitched at different levels. It can be descriptive. It can seek to analyse and interpret correlations, or it can seek to explain. The most important message for nursing is to strive towards an increased research mindedness; to use research findings as a facilitating tool, recognising its limitation yet capitalising on its strengths to improve practice and to delineate the unique discipline of nursing (Walsh and Ford, 1989). Research is still a word which is often shrouded in mystique and dissociated from the art of 'doing' by many practitioners. As a consequence, research is often seen as the pursuit of the 'highbrow' and this often causes the profession to revere certain persons and to accept their offerings as 'the bible' of truth (Clifton, 1992). Clifton, in his most illuminating article, warns against the tendencies which nurses display to 'pick heroes and follow them blindly'.

Research is not necessarily a daunting undertaking; small practical research questions that result from clinical interests and curiosity can yield very useful results. There are many research publications which can give practitioners a helping hand, for example Cormack (1991). In addition, expert help is available from various institutions such as the RCN Research Society, or the practitioner's local Department of General Practice, or Department of Nursing. The Strategy for Nursing actively encourages nurses to establish links with a recognised centre of research (Target 8) and to play an increasingly prominent part in ethical committees overseeing research (Target 9).

Local interest groups also provide peer support and a valuable research population. There is a wealth of research material to be found within such communities, the records they keep and the observations they make. These are resources which are relatively easily accessed without extensive additional amounts of time or money (Cox and West, 1986). So the type of research engaged in by nurses is not necessarily costly. Research reports appear in several of the popular nursing journals, although nurses should be encouraged to read more widely. Most clinicians are interested in applied research that can help them in their everyday practice, either in terms of evaluating consumer satisfaction or identifying consumer needs.

However, there is a need to be alert to the paradox of research during periods of economic constraint. At such times it is often seen as a luxury when, in reality, it is often at its most valuable because of its ability to increase cost-effectiveness (Perry and Jolley, 1991). Clearly, research has ethical, moral, practical, professional and educational implications for the future of nursing in general practice and the wider context of the PHCT. The nurse, in concert with other disciplines, should be willing to advocate for the patient where there is a real belief in the value of research and the contribution it could make towards the validation of professional standards by encouraging good practice and discouraging those practices which are found to be ineffective. Research is promoted by the Statutory Bodies; for example UKCC concludes that because nursing is a complex activity, intimately linked with the work of several other professions, 'Council should concentrate on the promotional and facilitatory aspects of its research function by ... encouraging and arranging multidisciplinary research activities to promote the concept and practice of partnership in clinical research' (UKCC, 1983).

Nursing in general practice provides a unique focus for research. There is an urgent need to document practice, objectively evaluate and describe the discipline base. Some examples of the research questions which need to be addressed include:

● What do nurses in general practice actually do, can they do, should they do ?
● How effective are they in what they do, for example in relation to the management of the asthmatic patient, or the monitoring of patients suffering from diabetes?
● How safe is clinical practice? For example, the aim of a small piece of research undertaken by a student as part of the course work on a recent practice nurse course was to measure the level of protection against hepatitis B within her peer group, to assess the main incidents of risk, and to make recommendations for the practice. The project revealed some interesting and useful findings.
● What are the continuing education needs of nurses in general practice? A piece of research completed by a practice nurse as part of a continuing education scheme asked 'Are practice nurses prepared for their role in the care of patients suffering from AIDS and/or HIV?' The aim was to assess the nurse's knowledge base, skills and attitudes, and to make recommendations for education and support networks.

The nurse can become involved in research in many ways. First and foremost is his/her willingness to question practice and by a commitment to the value of research. Other ways of making a contribution, or engaging in research include:

● Quality documentation and evaluation of nursing interventions.
● Audit within general practice, with due regard to the results.
● Interest in, and the ability to read and selectively apply research findings to inform practice.
● Responding to on-going research as a means of sharing information and developing research expertise.
● Participation in joint projects with colleagues who are more experienced in research.
● Engage in personal research, or if inexperienced, register on a course which includes research activities.
● Seek contact with and encourage other students who are developing research skills as part of their education and training, e.g. pre-registration nursing students (Project 2000, UKCC, 1986) and students who are preparing for the professional role in general practice.
● Promote the value of research through interest group networks, conferences.
● Push for the inclusion of multiprofessional research modules as part of all practice nurse courses and continuing education programmes.

Many readers will have listened to, or read of Lizbeth Hockey's account of her early days in the profession. She was always asking why, but was actively discouraged from such trivia. So she kept a small note book in her pocket and instead of asking why, she wrote her questions down on paper to be enjoyed later. She investigated numerous sources to find her answers and eventually she began to compare 'X' with 'Y' when she began to observe variations which were not immediately explainable. This was the beginning of a career in research and the insatiable desire to ask 'why'. Could this be you?

Summary

This chapter has considered a range of management processes and tools which also have relevance for a systematic approach to questioning practice. Some of the practical and ethical issues confronting the nurse in general practice during this period of unprecedented change have been opened for further debate as a means of promoting professional development. The overriding component of good management is the skilful deployment of resources; the essence of research is the validation of practice, thus contributing to quality care and professional accountability.

References

Anderson E, McFarlane J and Helton A (1986), Community-as-client: a model for practice. *Nursing Outlook*, **September/October**, pp. 220–224.

Armstrong M (1988), A *Handbook for Personnel Management and Practice*. London: Kogan Page.

Audit Commission for Local Authorities and the National Health Service in England and Wales (1992), *Homeward Bound: A New Course for Community Health*. London: HMSO.

Baliant E and Norell J S (eds) (1973), *Six Minutes for a Patient: Interactions in GP Consultations*. London: Tavistock.

Bowlden K J and Tackle B A (1989), *Practice Nurse Handbook*. London: Blackwell Scientific Publications.

Bradshaw P L (ed) (1989), Teaching and Assessing in Clinical Nursing Practice. London: Prentice Hall.

Briggs N J (1982), *Report of a Statewide Task Force on Nursing Competencies*. Wisconsin: W. K Kellogg Foundation.

Buckley G (1990), Auditing the organisation. In: Marinker M (ed) *Medical Audit in General Practice*. British Medical Journal, pp. 144–167.

Cox R C and West W L (1986), *Fundamentals of Research for Health Professionals*. Maryland, USA: Ramsco Publishing Co.

Clifton B (1992), Fighting hearsay is heresy. *Nursing Standard*, **6** (32), p. 45.

Cormack, D F S (1991), *The Research Process in Nursing*. London: Blackwell Scientific Publications.

Damant M (1990), *Report of the Review Group for the Education and Training for Practice Nursing 'The Challenges of Primary Health Care in the 1990s'*. London: (ENB).

DOE (PL 700) *Employment Legislation: Written Statement of Main Terms and Conditions of Employment*. London: DOE.

DOE (PL 919), *Guidance on the Employment Agencies Act 1973 and Regulations. Employment Agency Licensing Service Standards*. London: DOE.

DOH (1987), *Promoting Better Health*. London: DOH.

DOH (1989), *Working for Patients: A Review of the NHS*. London: HMSO.

DOH (1989), *Caring for People: A Review of Care in the Community*. London: HMSO.

DOH (1991), *The Patients' Charter*. London: HMSO.

DOH PL/CMO (89) 7 and PL/CNO (89) 10 and HC (77) 22, *Extending the Role of the Nurse*.

DOH Nursing Division (1990), *Nursing Prescribing: A Report of the Working Group*. London: DOH.

DOH HC (FP) (90) 8. *Health Service Development: Working for Patients. Medical Audit in the Family Practitioner Services*. London: DOH MED-H (Primary Care Services).

DOH and Welsh Office (1990), *Terms and Conditions for Doctors in General Practice*. The NHS (General Medical and Pharmaceutical Services) Regulations 1974 Schedules 1–3 amended. London: HMSO.

DOH Nursing Division (1986), *'Mix and Match': A Review of Nursing Skill Mix*. Report of the Steering Committee (chaired by Patsy Wright-Warren). London: DOH.

DOH Nursing Division (1989), *A Strategy for Nursing: A Report of the Steering Committee*. London: DOH.

Dingwall R (ed) (1983), *Managing Time Effectively*. London: The Granary Press.

Dixon P (1990), *Models of Clinical Management*. London: Institute of Health Service Management.

Eccles T (1977), Community Nurses and the Computer. *Queen's Nursing Journal*, **May**, pp. 391–392.

Greenfield S, Stilwell B and Drury M (1987), Practice nurses: social and occupational characteristics. *Journal of the Royal College of General Practitioners*, **37**(301), pp. 341–345.

Hall M and Hopkins R (1990), *NHS Management Executive: The Care Card. An Evaluation of the Exmouth Project*. London: HMSO.

Ham C (1990), *Holding on Whilst Letting Go*. London: King's Fund Project Paper No 86.

Hockey L (1966), *Feeling the Pulse*. London: Queen's Institute of District Nursing.

Hockey L (1968), *Care in the Balance*. London: Queen's Nursing Institute.

Hockey L (1972), *Use and Abuse*. London: Queen's Nursing Institute.

Hoffman W M and Wyly T J (1979), *The Work Ethic in Business*. Washington: Oelgeschlager, Gunn and Hain.

Hopkins R (1990), The Exeter Care Card: a CCP8-based global health care record for the United Kingdom's National Health Service (Editorial). *Journal of Medical Systems*, **14**(3), pp. 150–154.

Jeffree P (ed) (1990), *The Practice Nurse: Theory and Practice*. London: Chapman and Hall.

Kerrane L (1989), Staff appraisal and performance review. In: Dodwell M and Lathlean J (eds) *Management and Professional Development for Nurses*. Harper and Row, London: Lippincot Nursing Series.

MacFarlane J K (1970), *The Proper Study of the Nurse*. London: RCN Research Series.

Miller S J and Bryant W D (1965), A division of nursing labor, Community Studies Inc. In: DOH Nursing Division (1986), *'Mix and Match': A Review of Nursing Skill Mix*. London: HMSO.

Neuman B (1980), The Betty Neuman Health Care Systems Model – a total person approach to patients' problems. In: Riehl J and Roy C (eds) *Conceptual Models for Nursing Practice*. Appleton-Century-Croft, East Norwalk, CT.

Neuman, BM (ed) (1982), The Neuman System Model: Application to Nursing Education and Practice. East Norwalk, CT: Appleton-Century-Croft.

Nurses, Midwives and Health Visitors Act (1978 and 1992), London: HMSO.

Perry A and Jolley M (1991), *Nursing: a Knowledge Base for Practice*. London: Edward Arnold.

Pringle M (1990), Practice reports. In: Marinker M (ed) *Medical Audit in General Practice*. British Medical Journal, pp. 196–223.

Pyne R (1992), *Professional Discipline in Nursing, Midwifery and Health Visiting*. London: Blackwell Scientific Publications.

Reedy B L E, Philips P R and Newell D J (1976), Nurses and nursing in primary medical care in England. *British Medical Journal*, **2**, pp. 1304–1306.

Ross F (1988), Information sharing between patients, nurses and doctors: evaluation of a drug guide for older people in primary health care. *Recent Advances in Nursing*, **21**, London: Longman, pp. 159–185.

Ross F (1989), Doctor, nurse and patient knowledge of prescribed medication in primary care. *Public Health*, **103**, pp. 131–137.

Roy S (1991) In: *Report of the Working Group. Nursing in the Community*. London: North West Thames Regional Health Authority.

Royal College of Nursing (1991), *Professional Profile for Practice Nurses*. London: RCN.

Royal College of Nursing (1992), *Skill Mix and Reprofiling: A Guide for RCN Members*. London: RCN.

Secretary of State for Social Services (1987), *Promoting Better Health: The Government's Programme for Improving Primary Health Care*. London: HMSO.

Smith D (1972), *Nil by Mouth*. London: RCN Research Series.

Stockwell F (1976). *The Unpopular Patient*. London: RCN Research Series,.

Stilwell B (1982), The nurse practitioner at work. *Nursing Times*, **27 October**, pp. 1799–1803.

UKCC (1983), *Nursing Research: The Role of the UKCC*. London: UKCC.

UKCC (1986), *Project 2000: A New Preparation for Practice*. London: UKCC.

UKCC (1990), *Statement on Practice Nurses and Aspects of the New GP Contract*. London: UKCC.

UKCC (1992a), *The Code of Professional Conduct for the Nurse, Midwife and Health Visitor, 3rd edn.* (plus advisory statements). London: UKCC.

UKCC (1992b), *The Scope of Professional Practice for the Nurse, Midwife and Health Visitor*. London: UKCC.

Walsh M and Ford P (1989), *Nursing Rituals, Research and Rational Actions*. London: Butterworth–Heinemann.

Welsh National Board for Nursing, Midwifery and Health Visiting (1991), *Professional Profile: Cardiff*. London: WNB and Austen Cornish.

Whincup M (1982), *Legal Aspects of Medical and Nursing Service*. Kent: Ravenswood.

WHO (1978), *Health For All: Alma-Ata Declaration*. Geneva: WHO.

Wilkin D, Hallam I and Doggett A (1992), *Measures of Need and Outcome for Primary Health Care*. Oxford: Oxford University Press.

Wiseman J (1977), A nursing audit of basic care – 1. Occasional paper. *Nursing Times*, **73**(44).

7 Change and opportunities for nursing in general practice

7.1 The change process

Change is inevitable but offers the opportunity for development and progress. An important principle in the process of change is stability. The patient is still the prime consideration and general practice would not be general practice if nursing was not part of it. Further, although community nursing may develop in the future it will do so from its roots in existing practice.

Nurses in general practice often advance the argument that they effect change in the clinical setting. The authors have observed that course work undertaken by nurses attending educational programmes tends to support such assertions. For example, activities involving the preparation of a new protocol, or revision of an existing one, accompanied by a marketing plan for change, will show the extent to which an informed and skilful nurse can exert influence within the practice. Likewise, small projects such as audit, have the capacity to demonstrate the way in which nurses in general practice can question and systematically evaluate their practice and institute change. However, nurses along with their primary health care team colleagues are also increasingly experiencing rapid and continuing change for which they may feel ill-prepared.

Change can be suggested to be a fragile process and a source of stress. Stocking (1985) describes some factors which influence the process of change in a study of 22 innovations in the NHS. It appeared that factors other than what was actually being changed were as important, if not more important to the individuals involved. The degree of confidence invested in the people introducing the change was critical. For example where a new post is created and a member of the team is promoted, the degree of confidence in that person by other team members will be directly related to their perceived competence. In addition, individuals tend to reflect on the extent to which the change will affect their status, role and routines within the organisation. The acceptance or rejection of change by an individual appeared to be on intuitive grounds as well as the result of reasoning. The reaction of the group and attitudes towards the change from outside the group also influenced individuals. Clearly change is a group process and the implication of this for nurses in general practice has been discussed in relation to teamwork. The outcome of the change process may not only result in different methods of working, but the experience can also result in personal growth and professional development.

Several texts are available to assist the understanding of change and the ability to manage change creatively (Schurr and Turner, 1982). The ENB learning package 'Managing Change in Nursing Education' (1988) can be adapted easily and applied to the change process in practice settings. It gathers together accessible literature which is relevant and practical. Change will be a major challenge for nurses in general practice as the twentieth century draws to a close and the twenty-first century dawns. It would be helpful at this point to consider the opportunities for developing nursing in general practice. Are we considering practice nurses, or nurse practitioners? Is nursing in general practice a discrete area of community nursing or a separate discipline? There are no clear answers to these questions but the issues surrounding these questions are the substance of this chapter. **Figure 7.1** attempts to summarise the context in which opportunities for development will occur. Each issue will be examined separately.

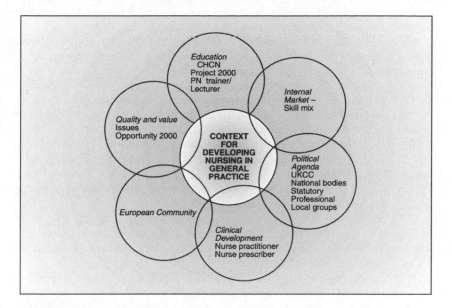

Figure 7.1 The context for potential developments.

7.2 The internal market

Opportunity to advance nursing in general practice can only be built on the knowledge of a framework for the delivery of health care.

Underpinning the emphasis on health services management is the framework of the internal market whereby contracts are agreed between the purchasing agent and the provider agent based, in principle, on needs assessment, and providing quality care.

Service specifications are set by the purchasing agent and are then negotiated with the provider of the services. The division between the two agents has come about by dividing the Health Authorities/Boards from the management and delivery of the provider services. A number of patterns have emerged, including the merging of Authorities (e.g. Family Health Services Authority with the District Health Authority) as joint purchasing agents, and the creation, or enhancement, of a separate purchasing authority as sole purchaser of primary health care services. Provider agents are the trusts and units of services within their own management structure. In principle, it is more important that whatever pattern is adopted, it is that which dictates policy and policy is not dictated by what is available.

This has brought management to a more localised focus – a sharper and more realistic accountability of the services provided. Standards can be set and monitored that are pertinent to the health care needs of a particular locality and meet the contractual requirements. The system of management also stimulates a degree of competition as the purchaser may have the choice of provider agents who themselves have to develop marketing skills to 'sell' their package of care. So what does nursing in general practice have to sell?

General Practice Fund holders have both a purchaser and provider role – both buying in services on a contractual basis and delivering services to the practice population. Fund holding is a partnership between GPs and patients, shifting power away from the consultant provider to the GP purchaser. Following detailed planning and data collection in the year prior to fund holding, financial resources are allocated from Regional Health Authority through the Family Health Service Authority. Under the NHS and Community Care Act 1990, FHSAs have responsibility for the day to day monitoring of fund expenditure but there is no direct accountability. Legislation is likely to be brought in which will make this clear. The commercialisation of health care has involved the appointment of business managers who provide support in data collection, strategic planning and contracting.

It can be seen that the structure whereby service specifications are developed and contracts negotiated between the purchaser and provider can be powerful frameworks to monitor standards and enhance patient care. An example of this is demonstrated in the following incident.

A general practitioner from a non-fund-holding practice referred a patient to the gynaecological department for an urgent appointment because of suspected ovarian cancer. The appointment was given for 3 weeks later. Turning to the Trust's service specifications he read that urgent GP referrals would be seen within 1 week. The person responsible for ensuring that standards were kept was named in the document. This person was telephoned and challenged and the patient was seen within 1 week.

7.3 Clinical development

7.3.1 Professional opportunities

While it has been suggested that changes in management can enhance patient care and the meeting of health care needs, there are also issues that potentially affect community nursing and in particular nursing in general practice. It will be increasingly important for nurses to identify clearly how they can determine and meet the health needs of the practice population.

From a purchasing perspective, if the purchaser does not appreciate the relevant nursing skills to provide effective health care, then the services bought in could be inappropriate. The agent may be more concerned with numbers and value for money rather than quality and select a cheaper option. It is a matter of concern that purchasing agents may not have a commitment for ensuring nursing advice as they develop service specifications.

From April 1993 GP Fund holders will be given a budget to purchase district nursing and health visiting services from community service units. It is possible that practice nurses could be employed on the same basis or alternatively they can become partners in the practice and independent contractors themselves determining and managing the nursing needs of the practice.

Alternatively, the FHSA could standardise terms and conditions whilst the professional contractual link between the nurse and GP is maintained. The budget for purchasing the district nursing and health visiting services will be based on the level of activity during the previous financial year, taking into account any anticipated changes and the cost of providing those services. For the first year there will be minimal opportunity for changes. However there can be more flexibility and negotiation after the first year.

There is concern that should GP fund holders become the employers of nursing services they will find it difficult to support statutory conditions of service, educational and professional needs as well as occurrences such as cover for annual leave and sickness. If nurses were to become partners they would need to negotiate adequate partnership agreements covering, for instance, profit sharing, pension and making contribution to the 24 hours of service provision. This may include undertaking night visits as part of an on call roster and arranging locum relief. The nurse partner would understand the roles and potential of community nursing to meet health care needs.

The appointment of nurse advisers and primary health care facilitators is intended to assist the development of nursing in general practice. A number of nurses in general practice have taken on these roles as part of their professional development, using their experience and skills to influence nursing in general practice across a health district. The facilitator role evolved from the Oxford prevention of heart attack and stroke project started in 1982 and is now a national facilitator development project under the directorship of Elaine Fullard. The role has developed from being solely concerned with audit to project development of health promotion activities, dissemination of good clinical practice, team development and bridge building/liaison. A number of facilitators have had joint appointments between FHSAs and District Health Authorities; their role tends towards that of provider.

The first nurse adviser to be appointed was to East Sussex FHSA in 1988. The post was specifically developed to address a wider remit than that of facilitator, not only influencing patient care and terms and conditions of service for nurses in general practice, but also contributing to the Authority's strategic planning and development. The nurse adviser was also expected to promote collaboration between Authorities to meet health needs and confirm the role of nursing in general practice as part of community nursing albeit with different employers. The role has developed much more towards that of purchasing – influencing policy and development and advising on service specifications.

Both roles continue to develop and there has been a degree of overlap. The patterns of management may see more division between the roles but both have the opportunity to ensure that nursing in general practice develops and is part of community nursing in order to meet health care needs.

7.3.2 Nurse prescribing

Responsibility for clinical decisions often results in the need for prescribing a treatment which is used only by the nurse, e.g. items for the treatment of leg ulcers such as hydrocolloids.

It is not appropriate for a professional to ask a GP to prescribe an item that he would not be using and has minimalist knowledge of its potential effects; it wastes GP time and may delay healing. It is therefore a positive move forward to professional accountability that there will be nurse prescribing using a Nurses' Formulary. The items prescribed will be those necessary for patient care and conditions for which the nurse is professionally responsible. Although initially only those nurses who are readily identifiable in the Professional Register by virtue of a health visiting or district nursing qualification will be prescribing, pressure is already being applied to extend the criteria to other groups of nurses who have comparable standard of professional education. There is obvious concern that legally and professionally the prescriber can be identified readily and be recognised to have validity. There are financial implications. The need to have an indicative prescribing budget allocated to community Units and Trusts and the issues surrounding that must not be underestimated.

For the nurse in general practice, it appears probable that the budget for nurse prescribing will be estimated with the GP's indicative prescribing budget – already for many in 1992 overspent. This raises a number of potential issues concerning her professional accountability and advancement as a nurse prescriber. The GP may be more concerned with the budget than with the professional issues and enhanced patient care. It is therefore essential that the nurse in general practice is able to demonstrate her financial accountability, her professional responsibility and acumen and her clinical assertiveness as a nurse in order to ensure that she can prescribe and advance her nursing practice and autonomy. At the time of writing financial implications have resulted in the postponement of nurse prescribing.

7.3.3 Shifts in health care within community nursing

The introductory chapter described developments within nursing in general practice within the context of community nursing as a whole. Changes continue to take place. The shift from hospital to community based care plus the increased resources of nursing within general practice have allowed district nursing (DN) services to focus their resources on the housebound ill person. The Children Act (1989) has emphasised the responsibilities of health visiting (HV). As a consequence, the opportunity for practice nursing (PN) to develop care for adults able to attend the surgery is enormous. It is enormous providing practice is underpinned by the appropriate level of clinical reasoning and a sound knowledge base. The shift in the present provision of nursing care in the community is illustrated in **Figure 7.2**.

One of the decisions for the future is the level of remuneration for carrying out delegated procedure (see discussion on skill mix in Chapter 6). There are also implications for education.

Figure 7.3 suggests three different levels of nursing taking place in general

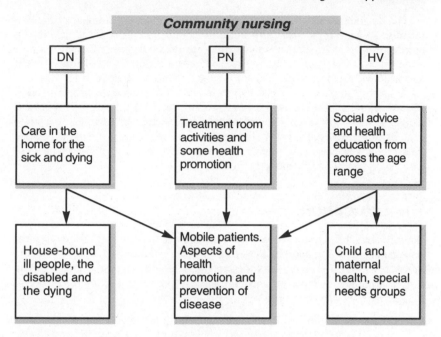

Figure 7.2 The shift within community nursing.

practice. The question for practice nursing is which route to follow or whether all three routes should be taken. The latter course of action allows flexibility to meet the needs of the practice population.

Taking the route towards managing the overall nursing care for patients could be to develop the role of nurse practitioner. This concept implies an independent practitioner working in collaboration with others. The collaboration is possible because of comparable levels of education and experience. It does not mean simply working by oneself. The district nursing and health visiting roles have the potential to, or indeed do, meet these criteria.

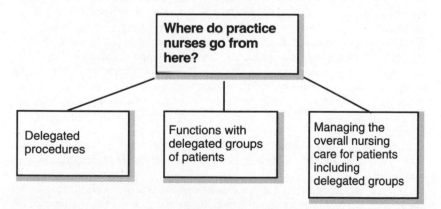

Figure 7.3 The development within practice nursing.

To continue the theme of autonomy, Stilwell offers an example of nursing initiative in general practice (Stilwell *et al.*, 1987). Her example of developing professional autonomy to meet the health needs of people where there was a lack of provision is well known. The project undertaken in South East Thames cited in Chapter 6 will do much to evaluate the potential of this autonomous role.

Another example of autonomous practice was with homeless people (Burke-Masters, 1986, 1988). This was a health service offered to people who were not registered with a GP. Such vulnerable groups are increasing in society – a prime example is the new age traveller. The people concerned may come to the practice if they are in one place long enough. However, they may fail to register with a GP and consequently will be deprived of health care.

7.4 Education

By 1993 the UKCC will have defined the standards to be met in relation to post-registration education and practice (PREPP). This includes community nursing practice – in itself a matter of wide consultation and discussion in 1992. The proposals, in general terms, received a positive response and in May 1992 Council reached the policy position as follows:

> The term 'community health care nurse' will be used in future ... to describe a registered nurse who has completed a specific post-registration preparation, which meets the Council's standards, in order to provide specialist nursing care in the community. This is *not* a proposal for a 'generic nurse', as a specialist preparation will be required for specific areas of practice, to reflect the diversity of need within the community.
>
> (Registrar's Letter, UKCC, 1992)

The preparation for this role will probably consist of a common core to be completed by all practitioners and then specialist practice-specific modules directed to an area of practice such as general practice. Currently, specific education for nurses in general practice is optional and therein lies the problem, for it is a mandatory requirement for district nurses and health visitors. For nurses in general practice this preparation should not now be optional but must be mandatory. Many educational institutions are developing their health visiting and district nursing programmes in anticipation of these changes, and in recognition of the needs of nursing in general practice. A system of credit accumulation has been developed in higher education in the UK. Previous appropriate learning and experience can frequently be accommodated within such a system. It appears likely that practitioners currently working in the community and who hold an appropriate qualification will be automatically recognised as Community Health Care Nurses.

These changes should bring together all nurses working in the community and demonstrate educationally that there is unity in the diversity of practice and the meeting of health care needs.

Three levels of function for nursing in general practice were described in **Figure 7.3**. The role of managing the overall care for patients could be developed further. **Table 7.1** illustrates different levels of performance that require different levels of educational preparation.

Table 7.1 Levels of expertise.

Novice	Experienced practitioner	Advanced practitioner	Expert practitioner
	Selects and uses research to inform practice, reads and selects from a range of nursing journals for personal professional development.	Critically evaluates and uses research to inform practice. Reads widely across disciplines.	Reads widely – across all disciplines.
	Ability to publish and make a positive contribution to the development of quality clinical practice.	Ability to publish and advance the professional knowledge and skills of others.	Ability to publish and to contribute new knowledge that expands the boundaries of quality professional practice.
	A facilitator of learning in the clinical area.	A teacher/assessor of practice and learning outcomes.	A teacher of theory and practice from first principles.
	A leader, supervisor and coordinator of a team of mixed skill professionals and helpers.	A manager of a clinical setting–functional or multidisciplinary.	An administrator of health care services.
	Reviews and maintains standards of nursing practice (audit) within a multiprofessional team.	Has executive functions and contributes to policy making.	Is concerned with policy making and evaluation.
	Participates in staff selection and the evaluation of job descriptions of posts within the team.	Sets and maintains standards of care and professional conduct. Institutes and manages the disciplinary process. Hires and fires. Advises on skill mix policies and monitors changing levels of acuity.	Able to influence directly fiscal policies for health. Hires and fires. Defines skill mix policies and institutes quality controls.
	Contributes to performance review and the identification of training needs.	Operates performance review, ratifies training provision and continuing education policies. Administers the training budget.	Negotiates contracts with educational establishments.Controls the training budget.
	Individually accountable for his/her own standard of practice and professional conduct.	Individually accountable for his/her own standard of practice and professional conduct.	Individually accountable for his/her own standard of practice and professional conduct.

NEWLY QUALIFIED NURSE

There are also changing levels of expertise at registration. Project 2000 establishes nurse registration at diploma level. However, looking at **Table 7.1**, it is clear that this is the starting point for nurses in general practice and where the teachers of nursing in general practice should be recruited and developed.

7.5 Quality and value issues

7.5.1 The named nurse

> The named nurse concept is a dimension of the greater responsiveness to the consumer ... It should be seen as an opportunity to apply a little imagination and creativity to patient care that is already well-rooted and flourishing.
>
> (Hancock, 1992)

For nursing in general practice, individual nurses tend to work on specific days and in similar clinics and the concept is not difficult to understand. The patient and nurse develop a partnership by virtue of each attending on the same days, or indeed that nurse may be the only one employed in the practice. However, the organisation will challenge the nurse in the need to ensure that patients are not only told but can read which nurse is working for that particular session. While it is usually clear which GP is in surgery, it is not usual to see which nurse is on duty.

Practice leaflets may indicate the nurses and their functions in the practice, but they are not usually individually identified. This may relate to the perceived potential for them to leave the practice and the practicalities of then changing the leaflet. The process will need to be worked through with the employing GP, but will enable the nurse to reiterate the significance of her role and position in general practice to meet health care needs. Some have already done this.

Another issue in relation to quality is retaining quality of provision where there is much change. Previous discussion has focused on changes in the working environment. But there can also be changes in the practice population such as housing developments that change the age structure of an area and consequently the health needs. Further groups, who themselves are very mobile, are inner city homeless and new age travellers who have already been mentioned. Both these groups have specific health needs which they bring to the practice, providing they register. General practice has always addressed problems of mental health and the specific needs of the patients and those who support them. People with learning difficulties are now becoming a more integral part of the community and they bring their special needs. Effective nursing within the multiprofessional team will involve recognising specific needs and making appropriate referrals. An underlying principle for practice is that it does not discriminate against people and, in sociological terms, marginalise them.

Nurses in general practice are in the main women, a historical perspective which opened the book. Links can be made between issues of quality in terms of effectiveness and efficiency and historical discrimination. The Department of Health has an active policy to increase the participation of women in the work force, but more important, to realise their full potential. Strategies are being developed within trusts and provider units to recognise staff potential and provide appropriate development. It can be argued that nurses working in general practice have potential that has yet to be realised fully. It is not cost-effective to under use, or ignore, valuable human resources. Indeed by 1992 it was estimated that there were 18–20,000 nurses in general practice and it is significant that in September 1992 the DOH had commissioned a practice nurse census. The census included requests for information about terms and conditions of service, qualifications, recordable or registerable education and clinical skills. The latter tended to reinforce the procedure oriented and delegated approach. However results will be disseminated in early 1993 and a second stage has been commissioned that will examine the roles and skills of practice nursing in more depth.

In the section on professional development brief mention was made of preparation for practice. Continuing education or continuous learning as part of everyday practice are central to maintaining quality of care. Learning that takes place in the workplace should not be undervalued, especially as this is within the context of the multiprofessional team and includes the patient. There is the opportunity of sharing experiences and deriving rapid benefit from feedback that allows alternative perspectives to be explored and considered. Within this scenario the opportunity to reflect through audit and research enhances practice further, adding a dimension of professional confidence and expertise. These activities can be formalised and documented via professional profiles. The emphasis is on what has been learned as a result of what has been done. The disadvantage of the traditional approach is that it concentrates on the activity, e.g. blood pressure measurement rather than the underlying clinical reasoning for carrying out the procedure.

Team meetings can serve a useful learning purpose, e.g. for the development of interpersonal and management skills. Knowledge can be gained and shared between the professions. Nurses can learn from doctors as doctors can learn from nurses. The addition of physiotherapists, occupational therapists and social workers to the team enhances the learning experience.

Earlier in the chapter it was suggested that it is not cost effective to under use or ignore valuable human resources. A system of performance review with an 'appropriate other' helps to prevent professional isolation. It also helps to identify skills that it is useful to strengthen further for the ultimate benefit of the practice population. An example of role development related to this could be a rural community where a nurse holds a nursing session in place of a previously GP run session in a branch surgery. The issue of the 'appropriate other' has been discussed in Chapter 3. Performance review is frequently linked to audit and therefore helps to identify what is considered to be the best use of scarce resources in the provision of comprehensive health care.

7.6 The European Community

The preceding discussion has assumed that nursing in general practice can be developed as nurses feel that it best meets patient needs. Much discussion has surrounded the issues of employer–employee power relationships. It is interesting to note that in other European countries the professional practice and education of nurses and therapists is largely controlled by doctors.

This suggests that nurses in general practice need to clarify their position quickly.

It is also useful to note that there are other differences between countries, for example how nursing is perceived, and there are differences in the roles and functions of nurses between member states. The nurse registered in general nursing has freedom of movement between member states based on a comparable educational structure, but there is no such protection for patients at post-registration level.

7.7 The political agenda

The Nurses and Midwives Act 1979 with the amendments made in 1992 was an opportunity for the profession to develop one voice for nursing. However in some respects the legislation might be seen to have continued the divisive element in nursing – namely nursing, midwifery and health visiting. It is interesting to note that the Royal Commission set up to examine the future of nursing, identified only two professional groups – nursing and midwifery (Briggs, 1972). An example to all professions at that time, was the demonstration of political strength and activity of health visitors. The Act has given and continues to give nursing the opportunity to develop professional autonomy and its independence from State control. The UKCC encourages all nurses, whose names are included in the Professional Register, to contribute actively to this process. An example of this is the UKCC's commitment to consult with the profession in advance of proposed changes regarding post registration and professional practice. The UKCC has reviewed the Code of Professional Conduct on three occasions because of the diversive nature of the changing context of nursing. Nurses have often initiated contact with the UKCC on a wide range of issues. They also responded to consultation exercises undertaken by UKCC. Nurses in general practice must join the debates and use the established political forums to safeguard the interests of the patients they serve. Indeed this has been done and is being done in several ways. Two Joint Committees with a UK orientation were set up by statute, namely the District Nursing Joint Committee and the Health Visiting Joint Committee. Practice nursing has had its own professional representation on the former for the past 3 years and on the Working Group advising on the community education and practice proposals. Nurses in general practice have also advised the Chief Nurse 1992 Task Force on primary care. The 1992 amendments to the Nurses, Midwives and Health Visitors Act of 1979 have brought about a different role for the UKCC and the Boards and changed the status of membership. The

UKCC is now the elected Body and practice nurses have presented themselves for election. Two areas of activity are implicit within this area and are:

● Preparation and commitment to stand for election.
● The motivation and understanding of colleagues to support the elected Member of Council.

Without these, the opportunity for practice nursing to be represented at UKCC could be negated.

Historical development of nursing in general practice has demonstrated its growth within the Royal College of Nursing. The Practice Nurse Association is said to be one of the most active membership groups. Nurses in general practice contribute and participate in the formulation of College policy and in particular to community health care nursing. At local levels, interest groups have formed Regional representation forums and have been active in creating links between FHSAs, Local Medical Committees and Institutes of Higher Education. It is this enthusiasm, political awareness and assertiveness of nurses in general practice that has provided the impetus for nursing in general practice to become established as a discrete area of practice and a potential force to be reckoned with politically.

Summary

This chapter has focused on change but for the management of change there needs to be a stabilising force. Health has always been central to primary care. Yet it is a dynamic concept which has changed due to environmental, scientific, technological and economic influences. However, nurses in general practice have shown evidence of being comfortable with changes associated with the promotion of health. It is important in a climate of change to look for stabilising factors. Nurses can do this by identifying central goals that they share with their patients and professional colleagues.

One goal is helping patients to make informed choices, as far as they are able, to achieve positive health. Facilitating independence can be influenced by helping patients to make choices. This could be another goal shared with professional colleagues.

This suggests returning to the basis of nursing and concentrating on practice. Various opportunities and challenges have been posed during the course of this chapter. One challenge concerned education. A stable base of general nurse training has allowed nurses in general practice to progress through a series of ad hoc training arrangements. The challenge for the future is to grasp more formalised educational opportunities as well as continuing their professional development through local initiatives. Further challenges have been posed which relate to the internal market and an increasing need to be politically aware. Nurses have been at the forefront of change in general practice and must continue to be so if the nursing needs of patients are to be met and the best uses made of finite resources.

References

Briggs A (1972), *Report of the Committee on Nursing*. London: HMSO.

Burke-Masters B (1986), The autonomous nurse practitioner. *Lance*t, **1**, p. 1266.

Burke-Masters B (1988), The nurse practitioner surgery. *Self Help*, **18**, pp. 22–23.

Children Act, (1989), London: HMSO.

English Nursing Board and Learning Materials Design (1988), *Managing Change in Nurse Education*. London: ENB.

Hancock C (1992), The named nurse concept. *Nursing Standard*, first published January 1992.

National Health Service and Community Care Act (1990), London: HMSO.

Schurr M and Turner J (1982), *Nursing – Image and Reality*. London: Hodder and Staughton.

Stilwell B, Greenfield S, Drury V W and Hull F M (1987), A nurse practitioner in general practice: working styles and pattern of consultation. *Journal of the Royal College of General Practitioners*, **37**, pp. 154–157.

Stocking B (1985), *Innovation and Inertia*. London: Nuffield Provincial Trust.

UKCC (1992), *Registrar's Letter – Proposals for the Future of Community Education and Practice – the Council's Policy Following Consultation*. London: UKCC.

Appendix 1: a genealogy of community nursing

COMMUNITY (GENERAL) NURSING

Selected aspects of change from:

PRE-PROFESSIONAL ERA: religious orders, philanthropists, self appointed 'wise women'

NIGHTINGALE

PRACTICE NURSING (PN)
- Doctor's lady

First PN employed

DISTRICT NURSING (DN)

Rathbone Liverpool
- First Nurse Mary Robinson (1862)
- First DN Course (1868)

Queen Victoria's jubilee Established QIDN (1887)
- 6 month course
- Roll of qualified DNs
- Inspected affiliated agencies

DN

OCCUPATIONAL HEALTH NURSING (OHN)

Coleman's of Norwich (1878)
- First nurse Philippa Flowerday
- OHN mornings, DN afternoon/ evenings

First OHN course
RCN London (1936)

Continued as a separate branch of nursing within the private sector

Developments in DN/HV education provided opportunities for shared initiatives (1980s)

National Boards established OHN Committees (1980s)

SCHOOL NURSING (SN)
- London (1892) SN morning, DN afternoon or evening duties

HEALTH VISITING (HV)

Health missioners (not nurses)
- Manchester and Salford (1862)
- Buckinghamshire Course (1891) Nightingale and De'Ath
First 3 HVs

Child life protection duties invested in HV

Huddersfield appointed medical officers to work as HVs

Royal Sanitary Institute
(Royal Society of Health in 1955)
Regulatory body for HV and SN
Courses, Examinations and Roll (1908)

SELECTED KEY FORCES:

Poor Law – less eligibility

Industrial revolution movement – from the land to towns

First population census (1801)

Proposed nurse training based on 'natural law' theory (1858)

Compulsory Education Laws (1870)

Baby farming – Mary Waters murders (1870)
Infant Life Protection Legislation (1872)

Registration of Births and Deaths Legislation (1874)

National Prevention of Cruelty to Children (NSPCC) formed (1884)

First school doctor (1890)
First school nurse (1892)

Boer War (1899–1902) – Grade 'C3' recruits

Population census (1901)
- Population had increased
- Continued move from the land to the towns

Shaftesbury's C18 factory reforms continue along with Chadwick's concern for the environment

Statutory regulation of midwifery practice (1902)

National Insurance Legislation for the employed (1911)

First World War (1914–1918)
- continued health deficits

Maternity and Child Welfare and Dental Services (M&CW Act 1918)
Ministry of Health formed (1919)

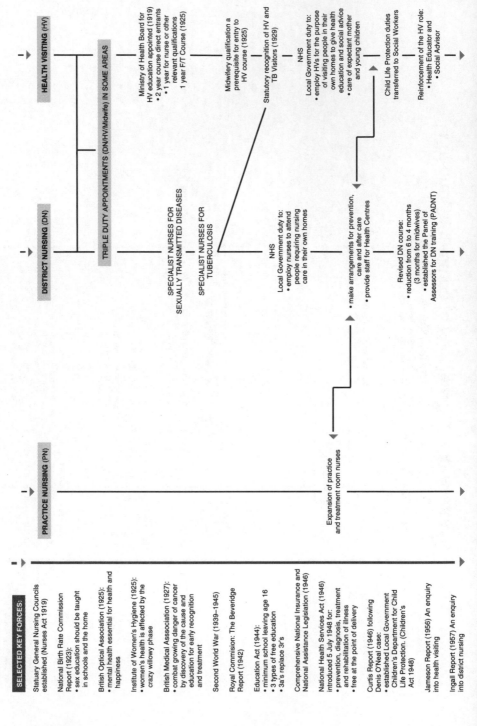

SELECTED KEY FORCES:

Statuary General Nursing Councils established (Nurses Act 1919)

National Birth Rate Commission Report (1923):
• sex education should be taught in schools and the home

British Optical Association (1925):
• mental health essential for health and happiness

Institute of Women's Hygiene (1925):
• women's health is affected by the crazy willowy phase

British Medical Asssociation (1927):
• combat growing danger of cancer by discovery of the cause and education for early recognition and treatment

Second World War (1939–1945)

Royal Commission: The Beveridge Report (1942)

Education Act (1944):
• minimum school leaving age 16
• 3 types of free education
• 3a's replace 3r's

Comprehensive National Insurance and National Assistance Legislation (1946)

National Health Services Act (1946) introduced 5 July 1948 for:
• prevention, diagnosis, treatment and rehabilitation of illness
• free at the point of delivery

Curtis Report (1946) following Denis O'Neal case:
• established Local Government Children's Department for Child Life Protection. (Children's Act 1948)

Jameson Report (1956) An enquiry into health visiting

Ingall Report (1957) An enquiry into district nursing

PRACTICE NURSING (PN)

Expansion of practice and treatment room nurses

DISTRICT NURSING (DN)

TRIPLE DUTY APPOINTMENTS (DN/HV/Midwife) IN SOME AREAS

SPECIALIST NURSES FOR SEXUALLY TRANSMITTED DISEASES

SPECIALIST NURSES FOR TUBERCULOSIS

NHS
Local Government duty to:
• employ nurses to attend people requiring nursing care in their own homes

• make arrangements for prevention, care and after care
• provide staff for Health Centres

Revised DN course:
• reduction from 6 to 4 months (3 months for midwives)
• established the Panel of Assessors for DN training (PADNT)

HEALTH VISITING (HV)

Ministry of Health Board for HV education appointed (1919)
• 2 year course direct entrants
• 1 year for nurse or other relevant qualifications
1 year F/T Course (1925)

Midwifery qualification a prerequisite for entry to HV course (1925)

Statutory recognition of HV and TB Visitors (1929)

NHS
Local Government duty to:
• employ HVs for the purpose of visiting people in their own homes to give health education and social advice
• care of expectant mother and young children

Child Life Protection duties transferred to Social Workers

Reinforcement of the HV role:
• Health Educator and
• Social Advisor

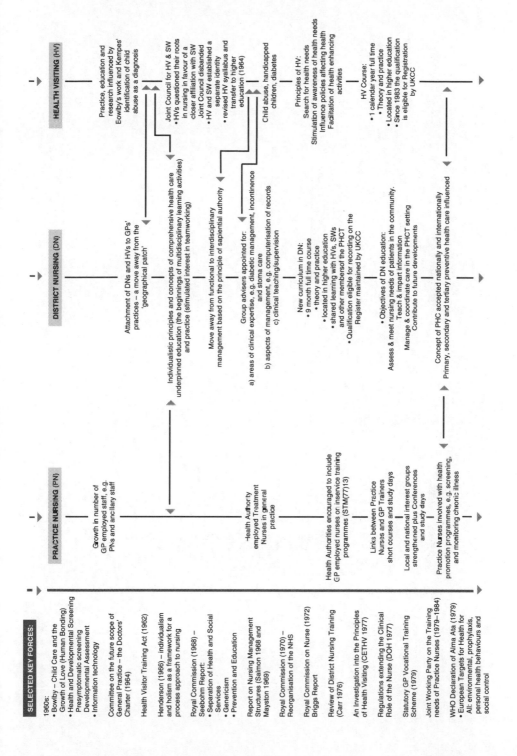

1960s:
- Bowlby – Child Care and the Growth of Love (Human Bonding)
- Health and Developmental Screening
  Presymptomatic screening
  Developmental Assessment
- Information technology

Committee on the future scope of General Practice – the Doctors' Charter (1964)

Health Visitor Training Act (1962)

Henderson (1966) – individualism and holism as a framework for a process approach to nursing

Royal Commission (1968) – Seebohm Report:
- Separation of Health and Social Services
- Genericism
- Prevention and Education

Report on Nursing Management Structures (Salmon 1968 and Mayston 1969)

Royal Commission (1970) – Reorganisation of the NHS

Royal Commission on Nurse (1972) Briggs Report

Review of District Nursing Training (Carr 1976)

An Investigation into the Principles of Health Visiting (CETHV 1977)

Regulations extending the Clinical Role of the Nurse (DOH 1977)

Statutory GP Vocational Training Scheme (1979)

Joint Working Party on the Training needs of Practice Nurses (1979–1984)

WHO Declaration of Alma Ata (1979)
- European Targets for Health for All: environmental, prophylaxis, personal health behaviours and social control

PRACTICE NURSING (PN)

Growth in number of GP employed staff, e.g. PNs and ancillary staff

-Health Authority employed Treatment Nurses in general practice

Health Authorities encouraged to include GP employed nurses or inservice training programmes (STM(77)13)

Links between Practice Nurses and GP Trainers short courses and study days

Local and national interest groups strengthened plus Conferences and study days

Practice Nurses involved with health promotion programmes, e.g. screening, and monitoring chronic illness

DISTRICT NURSING (DN)

Attachment of DNs and HVs to GPs' practices – a move away from the 'geographical patch'

Individualistic principles and concepts of comprehensive health care underpinned education (the beginnings of multidisciplinary learning activities) and practice (stimulated interest in teamworking)

Move away from functional to interdisciplinary management based on the principle of sapiential authority

Group advisers appointed for:
a) areas of clinical expertise, e.g. diabetic management, incontinence and stoma care
b) aspects of management, e.g. computerisation of records
c) clinical teaching/supervision

New curriculum in DN:
- 9 month full time course
  - theory and practice
  - located in higher education
  - shared learning with HVs, SWs and other members of the PHCT
- Qualification eligible for recording on the Register maintained by UKCC

- Objectives of DN education:
  Assess & meet nursing needs of patients in the community.
  Teach & impart information
  Manage & coordinate care in the PHCT setting
  Contribute to future developments

Concept of PHC accepted nationally and internationally
Primary, secondary and tertiary preventive health care influenced

HEALTH VISITING (HV)

Practice, education and research influenced by Eowlby's work and Kempes' identification of child abuse as a diagnosis

Joint Council for HV & SW
HVs questioned their roots in nursing in favour of a closer affiliation with SW
Joint Council disbanded
- HV and SW established a separate identity
- revised HV syallabus and transfer to higher education (1964)

Child abuse, handicapped children, diabetes

Principles of HV:
Search for health needs
Stimulation of awareness of health needs
Influence policies affecting health
Facilitation of health enhancing activities

HV Course:
- 1 calendar year full time
  - Theory and practice
- Located in higher education
- Since 1983 the qualification is eligible for Registration by UKCC

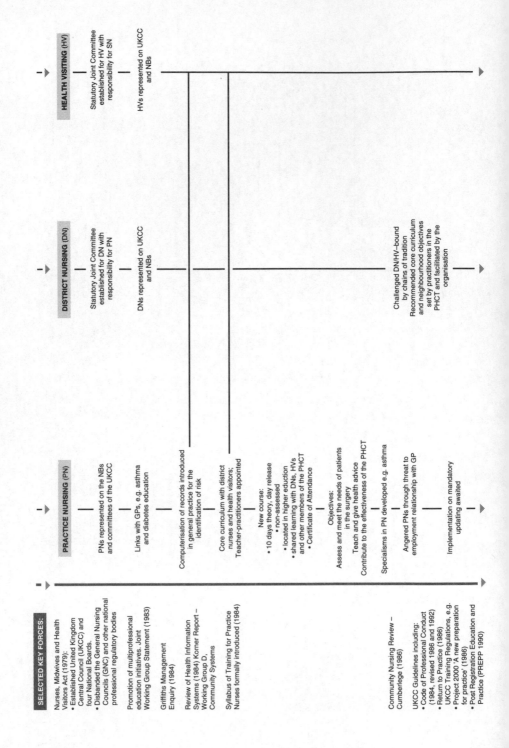

SELECTED KEY FORCES:

Nurses, Midwives and Health
Visitors Act (1979):
• Established United Kingdom
  Central Council (UKCC) and
  four National Boards.
• Disbanded the General Nursing
  Councils (GNC) and other national
  professional regulatory bodies

Promotion of multiprofessional
education initiatives. Joint
Working Group Statement (1983)

Griffiths Management
Enquiry (1984)

Review of Health Information
Systems (1984) Korner Report –
Working Group D,
Community Systems

Syllabus of Training for Practice
Nurses formally introduced (1984)

Community Nursing Review –
Cumberlege (1986)

UKCC Guidelines including:
• Code of Professional Conduct
  (1984, revised 1986 and 1992)
• Return to Practice (1986)
• UKCC Training Regulations, e.g.
• Project 2000 'A new preparation
  for practice' (1986)
• Post Registration Education and
  Practice (PREPP 1990)

PRACTICE NURSING (PN)

PNs represented on the NBs
and committees of the UKCC

Links with GPs, e.g. asthma
and diabetes education

Computerisation of records introduced
in general practice for the
identification of risk

Core curriculum with district
nurses and health visitors;
Teacher-practitioners appointed

New course:
• 10 days theory, day release
  • non-assessed
• located in higher eduction
• shared learning with DNs, HVs
  and other members of the PHCT
• Certificate of Attendance

Objectives:
Assess and meet the needs of patients
  in the surgery
Teach and give health advice
Contribute to the effectiveness of the PHCT

Specialisms in PN developed e.g. asthma

Angered PNs through threat to
employment relationship with GP

Implementation on mandatory
updating awaited

DISTRICT NURSING (DN)

Statutory Joint Committee
established for DN with
responsibility for PN

DNs represented on UKCC
and NBs

Challenged DN/HV–bound
by chains of tradition
Recommended core curriculum
and neighbourhood objectives
set by practitioners in the
PHCT and facilitated by the
organisation

HEALTH VISITING (HV)

Statutory Joint Committee
established for HV with
responsibility for SN

HVs represented on UKCC
and NBs

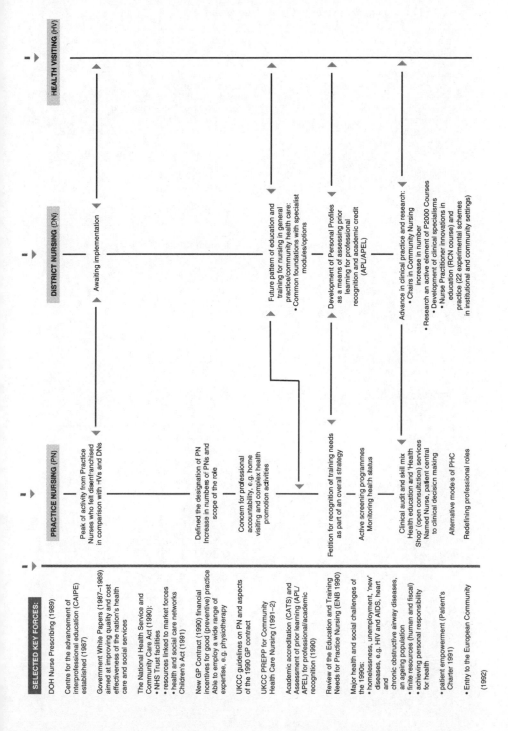

Index

Page numbers in *italics* refer to figures and tables

nurse *continued*
  practitioner experimental studies, 86
  prescribing, 94, 108
  registration, 112
  role in general practice, 21–4
  see also practice nurse
nurse–patient interactions, 34
Nurses' Formulary, 108
Nurses and Midwives Act (1979), 114
nursing
  aims, 51
  complementary role to medicine, 50
  documentation of practice, 51, 100
  documentation role, 59
  educational provision, 67
  European perceptions, 114
  expanding activities, 52–3
  extended role certificates of competence, 53
  extension of role, 54
  facilitation of integration of services, 65
  flexibility within general practice, 58
  framework, 50–1
  identity, *55*
  indicators, 88
  influence extent, 56
  intervention, 49
  organisational structure of services, 63
  patient needs perception in general
    practice, 58
  perceptions, 51, 114
  practice population needs, 87
  practices, *48–9*
  pre-registration training, 66
  professional autonomy development, 114
  range of activities, 49
  role in general practice, 49
  services outside hospital, 70
  sessions, 113
  utilisation of skills, 50
nursing care
  records, 90–1
  skill mix, 84
nutrition
  healing, 84
  health promotion, 84

occupational health nursing, *117*
occupational therapists, 35
occupational traits, practice nurse, 85
organisational models/structures, 63

paperless record systems, 81, 90
partnerships, 92
pathology, 12
patient
  advocacy, 57–8
  alliance, 39
  communication with professional, 39–40
  compliance, 39, 40–1, 70, 78, 94
  cooperation, 39
  coping assistance, 47
  dissatisfaction, 39
  empowerment, 57–8, 74, 96
  health promotion perspective, 78
  holding records, 59

patient *continued*
  implications of tests, 57
  information, 40
  informed choices, 80, 115
  lifestyle and nurse role, 50
  motivation, 77–8
  needs, 58
  needs assessment, 32–3
  nursing care, 47
  outcome, 35
  partnership with nurse, 112
  relationship quality with professional, 39
  role in decision making, 39–40
  satisfaction, 39–40
  value by nurses, 50, 96
patient care
  approaches, 47, *48*, 49–51
  enhancement by service specifications, 106
  framework, 51
  holistic, 57
  nursing framework, 50–1
  procedural framework, 49–50
peer
  assessment, 91
  review, 89
  support, 54, 67
  research, 99
performance review, 89, 95–6, 113
personality, barriers, 66
policy development, 58
political agenda, 114–15
Poor Law principle, 13
population
  expectations, 15
  expectations of health professionals, 14
  health needs, 60
  health status, 11
  trends, 11
  unrecognised health needs, 20
post-operative care, 31
post-registration education and practice
    project (PREPP), 88, 110
practice, developing, 42–3
practice nurse
  accountability, 52–3
  aims, 51
  assessment role, 32–3
  assistant status, 54
  autonomy, 17, 51, 85, 110, 114
  care provision for adults, 108
  census, 113
  chronic disorder management, 65
  clerical duties, 50
  clinical reasoning, 52, 66
  continuing education, 113
  contractual relationship with GP, 49
  debate, 51
  definition, 85
  designation, 84
  development, *109*
  diagnosis, 33
  documentation of patient care, 51
  education, 110, 113
  educational opportunity, 66
  employment, 17, 46
  employment relationship with GP, 81
  employment status, 92